SPINA BIFIDA
Problems and Management

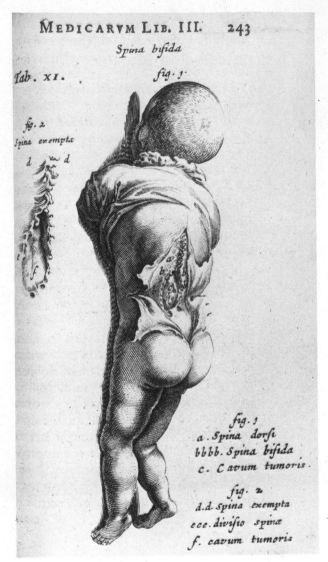

Frontispiece Dissection of a myelomeningocele by Nicolai Tulp (1652).

SPINA BIFIDA

Problems and Management

G. D. Stark

M.B., Ch.B., F.R.C.P.E., D.C.H., D.Obst., R.C.O.G.
Consultant Paediatrician, Royal Hospital for Sick Children, Edinburgh
Senior Lecturer, Department of Child Life and Health,
University of Edinburgh

BLACKWELL SCIENTIFIC PUBLICATIONS
OXFORD LONDON EDINBURGH MELBOURNE

© 1977 Blackwell Scientific Publications

Osney Mead, Oxford
8 John Street, London WC1N 2ES
9 Forrest Road, Edinburgh EH1 2QH
P.O. Box 9, North Balwyn, Victoria, Australia

British Library Cataloguing in Publication data
Stark, Gordon David
  Spina bifida: problems and management.
  Bibl.—Index.
  ISBN 0–632–00158–5
  1. Title
  618.9'27'3043   RJ496.S74
  Spina bifida

Distributed in the United States of America by
J. B. Lippincott Company, Philadelphia
and in Canada by
J. B. Lippincott Company of Canada Ltd, Toronto

Filmset by
Typesetting Services Ltd, Glasgow and Edinburgh
Printed in Great Britain by
T. & A. Constable Ltd.
Bound by
Hunter & Foulis Ltd.

Contents

PART 1
BASIC CONSIDERATIONS

PART 2
MYELOMENINGOCELE: CLINICAL PROBLEMS

PART 3
MYELOMENINGOCELE: MANAGEMENT

PART 4

MENINGOCELE, SPINA BIFIDA OCCULTA AND RELATED LESIONS

PART 5

THE FUTURE

Preface

Some explanation must be expected from a medical paediatrician who ventures to write a book on a condition for which treatment is predominantly surgical. In order to deal authoritatively and in depth with all aspects of spina bifida a group of surgical contributors would be required, as they are for management of the child. The aim of this book is, however, more modest. Although all the important problems of spina bifida are considered, emphasis has been placed on assessment and medical aspects of treatment and, in dealing with surgical treatment, on indications, limitations and complications rather than details of technique. It is intended primarily for the hospital or community paediatrician who is responsible for coordinating care of the affected child and requires a working knowledge of the important contributions which can be made by surgeons, therapists, social workers and many others. It is hoped, however, that for the surgeon it may provide a wider view of the child with spina bifida and of the way in which his contribution to management can be integrated with those of other members of a team with a common objective.

The idea of a combined spina bifida clinic in Edinburgh germinated more than a decade ago in the fertile mind of Dr T. T. S. Ingram. I am deeply indebted also to many colleagues who have played a major part not only in treating patients and supporting their families but in developing the concepts of management which I have described. In particular, I would like to thank Miss R. M. Mackay, Mr. F. H. Robarts and Mr. W. H. Bisset, paediatric surgeons; Professors J. I. P. James and D. H. Hamblen, orthopaedic surgeons; my neurosurgical colleague Mr. J. F. Shaw and consultant radiologist, Dr W. MacLeod. For an insight into non-medical aspects of spina bifida, I am grateful to Miss J. M. Mander, formerly neurological ward sister, to many social workers, psychologists and therapists in this hospital and to parents who have had to learn the hard way.

The following have generously given permission for reproduction of illustrations: Mr. W. J. W. Sharrard; Mr. R. B. Zachary; Drs W. J. Hamilton and H. W. Mossman; Messrs. Churchill Livingstone and the Editors of *Archives of Disease in Childhood* and *Developmental Medicine and Child Neurology*.

The manuscript was deciphered and typed by Mrs. E. Pay to whom I am most grateful.

To Anne Margot

Acknowledgements

I am grateful to the following publishers for their permission to reproduce illustrations.

Churchill Livingstone (Fig. 2.1 and Table 9.1)

Editor of *Archives of Disease in Childhood* (Figs. 5.1, 5.5, 5.6, 5.8, 5.9, 5.10, 5,11, 5,13, 15.3)

The Macmillan Press Ltd., and Drs Hamilton and Mossman (Fig. 2.7)

Editor of *Developmental Medicine and Child Neurology* (Figs. 6.2, 6.3 and 15.2(a)).

Editor of *Postgraduate Medical Journal,* Mr. R. B. Zachary and W. J. W. Sharrard (Fig. 17.1)

Editor of *Annals of Royal College of Surgeons, London* and Mr. W. J. W. Sharrard (Fig. 5.2)

PART 1

BASIC CONSIDERATIONS

The aim of the first three chapters is to clarify the terminology used and to present a brief introduction to the historical background, pathology, aetiology and incidence of the main varieties of spina bifida.

Chapter 1

Historical Introduction

Spina bifida has been recognized in skeletons found in north-eastern Morocco and estimated to have an age of almost 12 000 years (Ferembach, 1963). It was known to the ancient Greek and Arabian physicians who thought that the bony defect was due to the tumour. The term 'spina dorsi bifida' is, however, relatively recent, having been coined by Nicolai Tulp of Amsterdam in 1652. Professor Tulp, who is more familiar as the central figure of Rembrandt's painting, The Anatomy Lesson, appreciated from his dissection of six specimens that the protrusion in spina bifida could contain nerve tissue ('nervorum propagines tam varie per tumorem dispersas . . .'). His fellow-countryman Ruysch (1691) was, however, the first to make a clear distinction between paralytic and non-paralytic forms of spina bifida, i.e. myelomeningocele and meningocele. In 1761, in his great work *De sedibus et causis morborum*, Morgagni reported the association between lumbosacral spina bifida and both lower limb deformity and hydrocephalus.

In the nineteenth century came the unsurpassed classical descriptions of the morbid anatomy of various types of spina bifida. Professor Cleland of Glasgow studied specimens in the Hunterian Museum and in 1883 reported his findings. He described in detail the structure of a myelomeningocele and noted the frequent association of brainstem malformation, abnormalities of the axial skeleton and a post-anal dimple attached to the coccyx. Three years later, von Recklinghausen published his beautifully illustrated study which was based on dissection of 32 cases.

These anatomical studies intensified speculation about the morphogenesis of spina bifida which had already been a source of controversy for more than a century. Morgagni had postulated that the primary defect was occlusion of the central canal which led to 'hydrops' and rupture of the spinal cord and also to hydrocephalus. Béclard (1816) also favoured 'fetal dropsy' but attributed it, with less justification, to torsion of the umbilical cord and persistence of excessive fluid in the developing central nervous system. More mechanical views of causation were held by

1

Daresti (1877) who attributed the spinal defect to adhesions of the amnion to the back of the embryo and by Lebedeff (1881) who suggested that undue angulation of the spinal axis might prevent closure of the open neural groove.

Both Cleland and von Recklinghausen rejected the older theory of 'hydrops' and were convinced that the problem was one of failure of closure of the neural tube due to some disturbance of longitudinal growth of the embryo. As the fundamental defect, Cleland favoured overgrowth of neuroectoderm and von Recklinghausen advocated arrest of notochordal growth, concepts which are still widely supported.

The early writers were interested in spina bifida mainly as a fascinating experiment of nature. If they referred to treatment, as Morgagni did, it was only to warn against any kind of surgical intervention. In the nineteenth century, however, there were sporadic ventures in therapy. Newbigging (1834), for example, in his probationary essay for fellowship of the Royal College of Surgeons of Edinburgh, advocated an aggressive approach by puncture or ligation of the sac. Although he wrote of their 'happy results', these procedures were almost invariably fatal 'in consequence (according to Newbigging) of bad nursing'. In 1877, Morton, a Glasgow physician, described his method of treating myelomeningocele by injecting the sac with a mixture of iodine and glycerine. The initial results of this sclerosing therapy were encouraging but the later problems of hydrocephalus, infection and paraplegia proved insuperable.

One of the last surgical enthusiasts of this period was Sir John Fraser who in 1929 reported his experience of 191 cases of spina bifida cystica dealt with at the Royal Hospital for Sick Children, Edinburgh, between 1898 and 1923. No fewer than 131 children had been subjected to operation: 82 were discharged alive from hospital and, of 46 traced at follow-up, 30 were living. Surveying the results, Sir John concluded sadly: 'I wish I could say that the results were good: in a few cases, they might be so described – but the greater proportion were evidently crippled in body or in mind or both, and, as the records were gone through, one was inclined to say: 'Cui bono?' The first lesson of spina bifida had finally been learned: without the means to control hydrocephalus, treatment of the more serious forms of spina bifida was, for the most part, a lost cause.

A period of therapeutic nihilism ensued which contributed at least a clear picture of the natural history of untreated spina bifida. In a series of valuable papers, Laurence described the outcome of 381 cases of myelomeningocele born in South Wales at a time when surgical treatment was not practised. (Laurence, 1964, 1966; Laurence and Tew, 1971). At follow-up after 6–12 years, only 10 per cent of patients were still alive, and no fewer than 70 per cent were, by any standards, grossly handicapped. It was estimated that without surgical treatment, even ignoring stillbirths and first day deaths, only 1 in 7 would reach school age and 1 in 70 would be fit to attend a normal school (*Lancet*, 1969).

Towards the end of the 1950's the Spitz-Holter valve and ventriculo-atrial shunt were introduced and a new era in management of spina bifida began (Nulsen and Spitz, 1951; Pudenz *et al.*, 1957). For the first time, hydrocephalus was not a major barrier to treatment of spina bifida. As will be seen, however, with removal of this barrier, new problems have arisen and further barriers to effective treatment have been encountered.

Chapter 2

Classification, Pathology and Embryogenesis

Classification and Pathology

The ideal classification of spina bifida would have an embryological basis and, at the same time, be relevant to the clinical situation. Since such a classification is still elusive and this is intended as a practical guide, the conventional clinical classification will be employed throughout. An attempt will, however, be made later in this chapter to show how the more important lesions are determined during embryonic life.

The spinal cord is normally well protected by its immediate coverings: the pia mater which invests it closely, the arachnoid mater and the dural tube. It is suspended by the dentate ligaments in the spacious vertebral canal and cushioned by cerebrospinal fluid in the subarachnoid space. The secure bony canal is, in turn, covered by muscle, fascia and skin.

In spina bifida there is defective fusion of one or more posterior vertebral arches which may be accompanied by protrusion of the meninges, spinal cord or nerve roots beyond the normal limits of the spinal canal. There are two main varieties: spina bifida cystica and spina bifida occulta (Table 2.1 and Fig. 2.1).

TABLE 2.1. Classification of spina bifida.

Spina bifida cystica
    Myelomeningocele: open
                            closed
    Meningocele
Spina bifida occulta
    Isolated vertebral defect
    Associated anomaly (occult spinal dysraphism)

Spina Bifida Cystica

This term implies a cystic protrusion of the spinal cord and/or its coverings through a congenital defect in the posterior neural arches. It is not

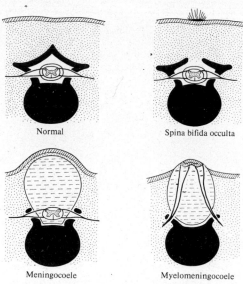

Normal   Spina bifida occulta

Meningocoele   Myelomeningocoele

FIG. 2.1. Classification of spina bifida cystica.

strictly accurate since, at birth, the lesion may be flat rather than pro-tuberant. Spina bifida cystica in turn encompasses two very different lesions: myelomeningocele and meningocele.

Myelomeningocele is the most serious variety of spina bifida. In it, there is a wide defect in the posterior neural arches: over several vertebral segments, the normal spines are absent and the everted pedicles and laminae are palpable well away from the midline. Through the bony defect, there is a protrusion of the meninges and neural tissue which is situated outside the vertebral canal. In the *open myelomeningocele* (Fig. 2.2) (synonyms myelocele, neurospinal dysraphism, rachischisis) the spinal cord is situated in the roof of the sac and takes the form of a flat neural plate at the upper end of which the central canal can usually be seen opening on to its surface. The nerve roots running from its ventral surface have a long course to the vertebral foramina and the roots of the cauda equina can often be seen at the lower end of the lesion through the thin bluish membrane (fused pia-arachnoid) which surrounds the neural plate. More peripherally, the lesion is joined by skin which is frequently thin and haemangiomatous. At the margin of the lesion, the dura fuses with the edge of the skin defect. The relative areas of exposed neural plate, membrane and skin vary considerably in different cases but the three elements can readily be distinguished by inspection of the lesion. This type of myelomeningocele is 'open' in two senses: the neural tissue is uncovered and it comprises an unclosed neural tube. By contrast, in

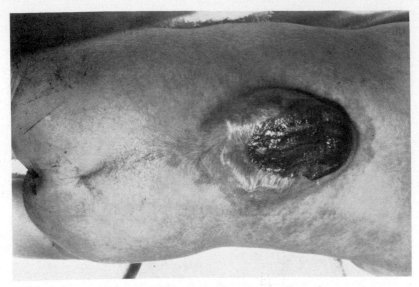

FIG. 2.2. Open thoracolumbar myelomeningocele.

the *closed myelomeningocele* (Fig. 2.3) although spinal cord and/or nerve roots are situated outside the vertebral canal, the neural tube is closed and the lesion is covered with a combination of skin and membrane. In the thoracic region, the closed myelomeningocele takes a characteristic form described as syringomyelocele in which there is cystic dilatation of the central canal of the cord whose thinned-out posterior wall protrudes through the bony defect and is covered only by a meningeal sac. As the vertebral arch defect is more localized in closed lesions, they tend to have a narrow base and pedunculated shape.

Surgical exploration and autopsy reveal more extensive abnormality of the spinal cord than the obvious myelomeningocele itself. Emery and Lendon (1973) in a study of 100 affected cords found dilatation of the central canal (hydromyelia) and/or syringomyelia cranial to the plaque in 43 per cent. Duplication of the cord (diplomyelia) was common at all levels but especially caudal to the plaque where it occurred to some extent in 52 per cent: separation of the two halves of the cord by a bony or cartilaginous spur arising from the vertebral body was, however, encountered in only a small proportion. In 9 per cent there was a hemimyelocele, i.e. the cord was split at the level of the plaque but only one-half involved in the lesion. Lipomas of the filum terminale, dura or leptomeninges are associated with myelomeningocele in as many as 75 per cent of cases (Emery and Lendon, 1969).

The upper end of the exposed neuroectodermal lesion coincides with the upper end of the mesodermal, i.e. vertebral lesion. The mesodermal lesion is, however, frequently more extensive distally than the neuro-

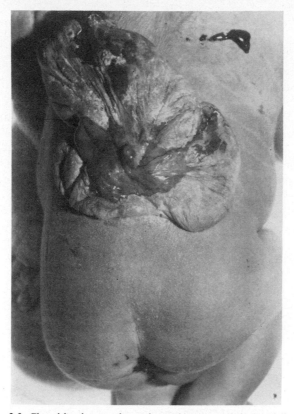

FIG. 2.3. Closed lumbar myelomeningocele, ruptured during delivery.

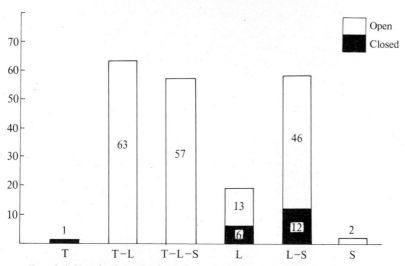

FIG. 2.4 Vertebral level of myelomeningocele. Distribution of 200 consecutive myelomeningoceles; 181 open, 19 closed; in relation to spinal level.

ectodermal lesion; in particular, if it involves the posterior arches of T12 or L1 it invariably extends throughout the vertebral column below that level (Barson, 1970a).

Myelomeningoceles vary enormously in size. Open lesions are usually between 4 and 10 cm and closed lesions between 2 and 6 cm in overall length. The incidence at different vertebral levels is shown in the histogram (Fig. 2.4). Two-thirds of open lesions involve the thoracolumbar junction, whereas closed lesions are situated entirely above or below this level.

Meningocele (Fig. 2.5). In the simple meningocele, the spinal cord is normal in situation and usually in structure. The bony defect is confined to a few vertebral segments and the protruding meningeal sac which has a narrow neck contains only CSF. The meningocele is covered by more or less intact skin. Like the closed myelomeningocele, the meningocele occurs in either the thoracic or lumbosacral regions and avoids the thoracolumbar junction.

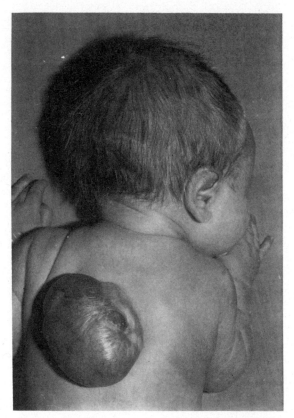

FIG. 2.5. Simple meningocele. (a) Neonatal appearance.

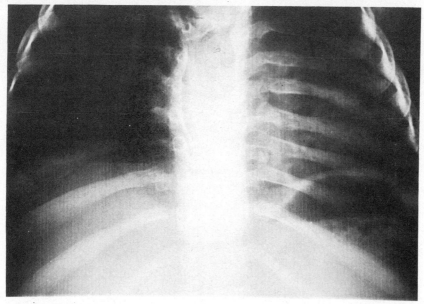

FIG. 2.5. Simple meningocele. (b) Posterior neural arch defect T4–8.

Spina Bifida Occulta

In spina bifida occulta, there is simply failure of fusion of one or more posterior vertebral arches, usually in the lumbosacral region. The defect may consist of a narrow oblique slit between the laminae or a wider palpable gap. It is 'occult' in the sense that it may be evident only on radiological examination (Fig. 2.6). There is no defect in the other coverings of the spinal cord and cauda equina which are situated normally in the vertebral canal.

It should be noted that, in the first year of life, when the posterior neural arches are not completely fused, spina bifida occulta is of little significance. Furthermore, there is evidence that an isolated defect limited to a single vertebra (usually L5 or S1) can safely be regarded as a normal variation (Laurence, Bligh and Evans, 1968).

A small proportion of patients have, in addition to the vertebral arch defect, a tell-tale lesion in the overlying skin or subcutaneous tissue. The lesions involved, including tufts of hair, naevi and lipomata will be considered in detail in Chapter 21. In a still smaller minority, an associated intraspinal anomaly is present and may lead to a neurological deficit. These intraspinal lesions, often referred to collectively as 'occult spinal dysraphism' have been described in detail by James and Lassman (1962); Dubowitz, Lorber and Zachary (1965) and by Till (1969). The more important lesions will now be outlined.

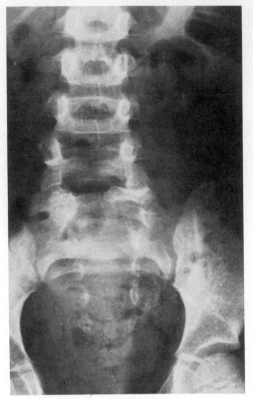

FIG. 2.6. Spina bifida occulta: narrow defect in L5 spine and wider defect in laminae of sacrum.

Low conus medullaris. In this condition, the spinal cord, which usually terminates at the third lumbar vertebra at birth, is elongated so that the conus is situated in the upper sacral region. The short filum terminale may be abnormally thick.

Diastematomyelia. Diplomyelia is simply division of the spinal cord into two halves which usually unite at a lower level and are enclosed in a single dural tube. In diastematomyelia, however, the half-cords are in separate dural tubes and there is some kind of septum between them representing an attempt to form a double spinal cord. The septum, which is attached to the vertebral body in front and to its laminae behind may be fibrous, cartilaginous or bony. Although usually a slender spur, it can occasionally take the form of a massive buttress of bone (Sedzimir and Roberts, 1973). In diastematomyelia, there may be hypoplasia or dysplasia of one-half of the lumbosacral spinal cord.

Hydromyelia. Dilatation of the central canal may be associated with spina bifida occulta as well as with myelomeningocele. It is commonly found proximal to a diastematomyelia and, if localized, may form a cyst capable of exerting pressure on the spinal cord (Lassman *et al.,* 1968).

Intraspinal lipoma. Lipomata of the kind which may accompany myelo-meningocele also occur in spina bifida occulta. They may be circum-scribed lesions of the dura or filum terminale. Of greater clinical importance, however, are fibrolipomatous masses involving the pia-arachnoid and attached, often inextricably, to a low conus medullaris and associated nerve roots. They may be connected to a larger sub-cutaneous lipoma by a fibrous stalk which passes through the vertebral arch defect. Histologically, they are not teratomatous but made up largely of normal adipose tissue.

Dermal sinus and dermoid cyst. A cutaneous sinus in the midline of the lumbar region may communicate directly through the neural arch defect with the spinal theca to form a neurocutaneous fistula. It may, however, be represented by a thin fibrous band attaching the cord or dura to subcutaneous tissues or by an intraspinal dermoid cyst.

Sacral extradural cyst. This lesion is a cyst arising from the tip of the spinal theca and situated posterior to the sacral nerve roots. As it is usually in communication with the subarachnoid space it could probably be more accurately described as an intrasacral meningocele.

Multiple Lesions

In 5 per cent of patients with spina bifida cystica, there is more than one spinal lesion. The second lesion is usually a stigma of spina bifida occulta such as a sacral dimple (an association noted by Cleland in 1883). Less commonly there may be two separate meningoceles and very rarely, three distinct lesions as in the patient described by Tryfonas (1973). The association of different types of spina bifida in the same patient suggests a common aetiological factor.

Normal and Abnormal Spinal Cord Development

Before considering the pathogenesis of various types of spina bifida, normal embryological development of the spinal cord will be outlined. For a more detailed account, the reader is referred to Lemire (1974) and standard embryological texts such as Arey (1965) and Hamilton and Mossman (1972).

Normal Spinal Cord Development

There are three more or less distinct and successive phases in spinal cord development: closure of the neural tube, canalization of the caudal cell mass and development of the coverings of the spinal cord.

Closure of the neural tube (Neurulation). The first stage in neural tube formation is differentiation of the pseudostratified cells of the neural plate from ectoderm. Induction of the neural plate which appears to depend on the influence of the underlying notochordal mesoderm takes place at 18 days of gestation. By 20 days, the neural plate has developed folds between which lies the open neural groove. The precise mechanism of folding is uncertain. There is evidence that it is, in part, intrinsic in the neural plate and, in part, dependent on some humoral influence from mesoderm.

At 22 days, when the embryo has 3 somites, the neural folds begin to close over the neural groove and fuse together. Fusion begins in the cervical region and proceeds in 'zipper' fashion towards each end of the embryo. The areas of the neural groove awaiting closure are termed the cranial and caudal neuropores – openings which are highly relevant to development of anencephaly and open myelomeningocele respectively. Closure of the neural tube takes only 4 days: the caudal neuropore closes at 24 days (15 somites) and the caudal neuropore at 26 days (25 somites). The cranial neuropore is at the level of what will be the hypothalamus and the caudal neuropore at the L1–2 intervertebral disc.

Following closure of the neural tube, its cells undergo rapid division and daughter cells migrate to form the main elements of the spinal cord and the motor axones of peripheral nerves. The cells which had previously lain at the margin of the neural plate on either side, come with closure to form a single column between the dorsal aspect of the neural tube and the overlying ectoderm. The cells of this 'neural crest' later migrate to form the posterior root ganglia, their axones and peripheral cells of the autonomic nervous system. At the same time, the notochord, previously in contact with the ventral aspect of the neural tube separates from it.

Canalization of the caudal cell mass. The process of neurulation accounts for development of the neural tube only down to the level of the first lumbar vertebra. Below this level, it differentiates from the caudal cell mass or tail bud which gives rise to many other important structures, including the kidneys. The neural tube emerging from the caudal cell mass differs from that formed by neurulation in that, from the beginning, it is covered by surface ectoderm; in other words, there is never an open neural tube below the caudal neuropore.

At 26–28 days gestation, vacuoles appear in the caudal cell mass and

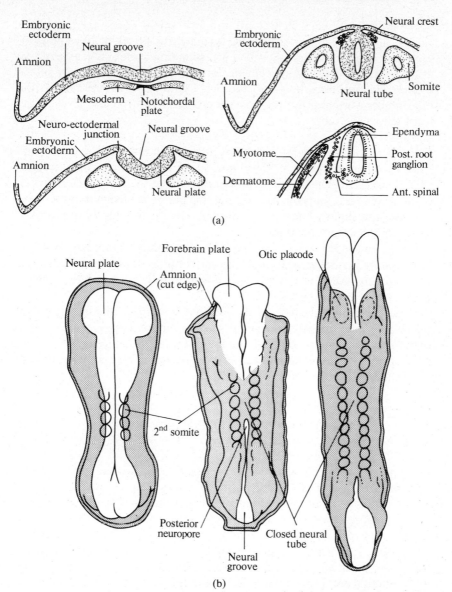

Fig. 2.7. Formation and closure of the neural tube. (a) In coronal section. (b) Dorsal surface.

gradually coalesce to form a central canal which becomes continuous with that of the more cranial neural tube. Much of the distal neural tube formed by canalization subsequently undergoes necrosis and atrophy and is finally represented by the filum terminale.

As a result of regression of the distal neural tube and the relatively faster growth of the vertebral column, the spinal cord recedes up the spinal canal as gestation proceeds. In the early stages of development, each cord segment is opposite the corresponding vertebral segment, e.g. at 60 days, the first sacral segment corresponds to the first part of the sacrum. By full term, however, the first sacral nerve is adjacent to the first lumbar vertebra and the spinal cord terminates at the level of the third lumbar vertebra.

Development of coverings of the spinal cord. Appearance of the primordial spinal cord is followed by development of its coverings in a cranial-caudal direction. The meninges differentiate from the loose mesenchymal tissue which surrounds the neural tube, the pia mater from about 40 days and the dura slightly later. It is, however, only much later that the arachnoid separates from the dura.

By the time that neurulation and canalization are complete at 45–50 days gestation, chondrification of the vertebral bodies and their posterior arches is advanced. The arches are, however, still bifid and the spinous processes have not appeared.

If, in experimental animals, the embryonic neural tube is extirpated, the vertebral arches fail to develop. Just as differentiation of the neural plate and neurulation depend on mesodermal influence, so, in turn, development of the vertebral arches and the size of the spinal canal are determined by the neural tube.

Embryogenesis of Spina Bifida

Although Morgagni's idea of rupture of the neural tube still finds occasional support, e.g. Gardner (1961), it is generally accepted that *open myelomeningocele* results from failure of closure of the caudal neuropore. The mechanism of 'non-closure' is, however, more controversial. Overgrowth of neural tissue has often been noted in the region of the myelomeningocele and has led to the theory that it could be the primary cause of eversion and non-closure of the neural folds. It can, however, also be argued that neural overgrowth is secondary to failure of closure. Abnormal vasculature at the site of the myelomeningocele could also be an effect as well as a cause of the neural tube defect. In view of the fundamental role of mesoderm in induction of the neural plate and in neurulation, some primary abnormality in the somites is yet another possibility.

The occurrence of *closed myelomeningocele* in the lumbosacral region reflects abnormality of the later process of canalization of the caudal cell mass. As has been noted, there is a preponderance of closed lesions in the distal cord which does not normally go through an open-tube stage. A variety of other abnormalities including *lipomata* and *myelodysplasia* can arise from failure of normal differentiation of the neural tube and related structures from the totipotent cells of the tailbud. Unrestrained development of this caudal cell mass can lead to a *teratoma* and arrest of development to *sacral agenesis*.

Failure of closure of the neural tube is followed by failure of vertebral arch formation. An isolated vertebral arch defect, i.e. *spina bifida occulta*, can be expected if deviation from normal development occurs later than 60 days. *Simple meningocele* may develop even later from protrusion of the dura-arachnoid through the defective vertebral arches.

TABLE 2.2. Embryogenesis of spina bifida.

Normal Process	Age	Result of Failure
Closure of caudal neuropore	26 days	open myelomeningocele
Canalization of tail-bud	26–30 days	{ closed myelomeningocele; occult spinal dysraphism
Early development of dura and pia	40 days	
Closure of posterior vertebral arches	60 days→	{ spina bifida occulta ? meningocele

Since, as already mentioned, the notochord is responsible for induction of the neural tube, it is conceivable that *diplomyelia* could result from a longitudinal split in the notochord. As the notochord is also involved in development of the vertebral bodies and intervertebral discs, a split notochord might be responsible for another related group of malformations (Bremer *et al.*, 1952; Bentley and Smith, 1960). Among these is *anterior spina bifida* in which there is a defect between two hemivertebrae and *diastematomyelia* with a bony spur formed by fusion of the medial pedicles of the hemivertebrae. Development of a communication through the notochordal defect between the entoderm of the yolk sac and the ectoderm of the amnion is thought to be the cause of *neurenteric cysts* and related lesions.

Chapter 3

Incidence and Aetiology

Spina Bifida Cystica

Incidence

As perinatal, neonatal and infant mortality rates progressively fall, congenital malformations loom larger as a cause of death in infancy. They account for almost 20 per cent of perinatal deaths in the United Kingdom (Butler and Bonham, 1963) and for an even higher proportion of chronic handicap in childhood. Among major congenital malformations, those of the central nervous system are not only the most damaging but the most frequent. In the U.K., the overall incidence of spina bifida cystica is of the order of 2·5 per thousand births which means that more than 2000 affected infants are born every year. While many paediatric units are now handling 50–100 new patients per annum, it is worth noting that the average family doctor could count on one hand the number of patients with spina bifida he will encounter in a lifetime of practice.

As shown in Table 3.1, there is considerable variation in the incidence of spina bifida cystica in different countries. Moreover, even within a small country such as the U.K., there are striking regional differences in incidence which falls steadily as one moves from the north-west of Ireland and Scotland to the south-east of England.

It should be noted that the figures quoted include stillbirths. In 1966, Knox estimated that one-quarter of affected infants were stillborn, but with increasing clinical interest and development of facilities for treatment, the proportion registered as 'stillborn' has fallen considerably. The reported figures for incidence are, of course, based on ascertainment at birth. There is, however, evidence that the incidence of neural tube malformations in embryonic life is substantially higher. In a Japanese study, for instance, myelomeningocele was found 13 times more often in abortion specimens than in full-term infants (Nishimura *et al.,* 1966). The statistics for spina bifida cystica include both myelomeningoceles

16

TABLE 3.1. Geographical variation in incidence of spina bifida cystica.

Place	Incidence per 1000 total births	Reference
Belfast	4·5	Elwood and Nevin, 1973
Dublin	4·2	Coffey and Jessop, 1957
South Wales	4·1	Laurence, Carter and David, 1968
Liverpool	3·5	Smithells and Chinn, 1965
Edinburgh	3·2	Nelson and Forfar, 1969
Birmingham	2·5	Leck et al., 1968
Sheffield	2·2	Lorber, 1969a
Budapest	1·9	Czeizel and Révész, 1970
U.S.A. (Teaching Centres)	1·2	O'Hare, 1958
Boston	1·3	Naggan and MacMahon, 1967
Melbourne	0·8	Stevenson et al., 1966
Israel	0·7	Halevi, 1967
Calcutta	0·5 ⎱	Stevenson et al., 1966
Singapore	0·4 ⎰	
Hiroshima and Nagasaki	0·3	Neel, 1958
Lagos	0·2	Lesi, 1968
Bogota	0·1	Stevenson et al., 1966

and simple meningoceles: in most series, however, the latter unfortunately account for no more than 10 per cent.

Aetiology

There is general agreement that, as for other major malformations, the aetiology of spina bifida cystica is multifactorial. While genetic factors appear to be involved, they may operate only by predisposing the embryo to the effect of some environmental influence during the first month of intrauterine life. The evidence for both genetic and environmental factors will be briefly reviewed.

Genetic Factors

In the U.K., it has been estimated that the heritability of spina bifida is between 50 and 60 per cent, i.e. genetic factors are at least as important as others in causation (Carter, 1974).

Spina bifida is recognized as one of the few malformations which are commoner in the female. The sex difference is, however, must less than in anencephaly and the ratio of females to males is little more than 1·2.

As noted in Table 3.1, there are large variations between different parts of the world and there is evidence that this racial variation is genetically determined. In Boston, for example, the incidence of spina bifida cystica in second and third generation immigrants still closely reflects that in their country of origin: for those of Irish Catholic origin it is 1·6 and for Jews 0·37 per thousand births (Naggan and McMahon, 1967). In the common environment of Birmingham, Leck (1969) found that the combined spina bifida and anencephaly rate was 5·8 per 1000 when both parents were Irish, compared with 5·4 for Indians and Pakistanis, 3·5 for British and 1·1 for West Indians. In several studies, Negroes and Japanese have been shown to have a low incidence even after emigration to areas of high incidence.

Consanguinity increases the risk of neural tube malformations and in the U.K. the recurrence rate is increased to 1 in 20 when one child has been affected and 1 in 8 after the birth of two affected children (Lorber, 1965; Carter and Roberts, 1967).

Although Lorber (1965) postulated that spina bifida might be due to a single autosomal recessive gene, the low recurrence rate in siblings and the slowly accumulating evidence of some risk to the offspring of patients are against it. The bulk of evidence at present suggests that predisposition to spina bifida depends on the combined action of a number of genes, i.e. polygenic inheritance.

The strongest evidence that genetic factors are not the whole story is the fact that monozygous twins not only may be but almost invariably are discordant for spina bifida (Laurence, Carter and David, 1968).

Environmental Factors

In animals, spina bifida can be induced by tampering with the intra-uterine environment in a variety of ways such as irradiation, administration of salicylates, Trypan blue or excessive amounts of vitamin A. In human beings, it is known that aminopterin can cause neural tube defects (Thiersch, 1952) but there is no evidence to incriminate more widely used drugs. Furthermore, Chadd *et al.*, (1970) found no elevation of IgM levels in cord blood to suggest intrauterine infection as a cause.

The evidence for environmental factors in the aetiology of spina bifida is, for the most part, of an indirect epidemiological nature. While international variation is in favour of a racial or genetic factor, striking regional differences within a small country point rather to an extrinsic factor. Such regional variation has been reported in South Wales where the incidence of spina bifida in the mining valleys is almost twice that in the coastal plain around Cardiff (Laurence *et al.*, 1968; Richards *et al.*, 1972).

In many areas, including Scotland, a significant difference in social class incidence has been noted, the highest rates occurring in the lower socioeconomic classes (Edwards, 1958). In most large surveys and even in clinical practice seasonal variation is apparent with an excess of affected infants in the winter months especially January and February suggesting that conceptions in March to May are at increased risk. Secular changes such as the decline in incidence in England and Wales between 1961 and 1968 and the rise from 1968 to 1971 would also suggest an environmental effect (Carter, 1974). Moreover, the incidence of spina bifida has a U-shaped distribution in relation to both maternal age and birth rank (Record and McKeown, 1249; Smithells and Chinn, 1965).

Despite compelling evidence for an environmental trigger which determines development of spina bifida in a genetically predisposed embryo, its precise nature remains elusive. Although it may well be secondary, a consistent inverse relationship has been found between hardness of water supply and neural tube malformations in England and Wales (Lowe *et al.*, 1971). More specific dietary factors have recently attracted attention. In 1972, Renwick propounded his much publicized hypothesis that anencephaly and spina bifida could be prevented in the U.K. by avoidance of potatoes in early pregnancy. Subsequent more critical studies have, however, largely exonerated the potato, blighted or otherwise, in causation of these malformations (*British Medical Journal*, 1972). Knox (1972) has listed certain foods including nitrite-cured corned beef and canned peas treated with magnesium salts which could be incriminated in anencephaly and other authors have considered the possible role of deficiency of zinc or folic acid in early pregnancy.

Spina Bifida Occulta

Incidence

From surveys of spina bifida occulta involving either radiological or postmortem examination there is general agreement that it is a very common lesion, but there is wide variation in reported incidence. Willis (1931) found it in 5 per cent of 1500 anatomical specimens and Karlin (1935) in no fewer than 54 per cent in a radiological study. Perhaps the main reason for such variation is the differing age structures of the series reported. It is now well known that spina bifida occulta is particularly common in children. It has been shown in Japan that the 5th lumbar spine is bifid in 16·1 per cent of children aged 7–8 years but in only 2·2 per cent of adults; the first sacral spine is bifid in 51·6 per cent of 7–8 year-olds and 26·4 per cent of adults (Sutow and Pryde, 1956).

Of greater importance, however, is the incidence of spina bifida occulta with neurological involvement ('occult spinal dysraphism'). Anderson's (1968) study suggests that it is about 15 per cent of the incidence of myelomeningocele.

Aetiology

As uncomplicated spina bifida occulta limited to either the 5th lumbar or 1st sacral vertebra can safely be regarded as a normal variant, consideration of its aetiology is irrelevant.

More extensive vertebral involvement accompanied by the potentially damaging lesions described in Chapter 2 is commoner in girls and can be placed at the opposite end of the pathological spectrum of spina bifida from open myelomeningocele. Evidence for this includes the common association of lesions such as lipoma and diastematomyelia with spina bifida cystica. Furthermore, parents and siblings of children with spina bifida cystica have an increased incidence of spina bifida occulta involving more than one spine (Laurence, Bligh and Evans, 1968). Although little research has been done on its aetiology, it is likely that the same combination of polygenic inheritance and environmental factors are involved as in spina bifida cystica.

PART 2

MYELOMENINGOCELE: CLINICAL PROBLEMS

Optimal management of the child with a myelomeningocele depends on a clear understanding of the basic clinical problems. Before considering management, therefore, the fundamental structural and functional defects will be reviewed.

The effects of a myelomeningocele are both profound and far-reaching. The most obvious is the *open wound* on the child's back. The most disabling is the *effect on the spinal cord* which in 95 per cent encompasses some degree of paralysis of lower limbs, bladder and bowel. To these are often added the problems of *associated malformations* and *secondary complications* which may greatly increase the child's initial load of disability.

Chapter 4

Immediate Neonatal Problems

The life of the child with myelomeningocele commonly begins with a difficult delivery. Malpresentation, forceps delivery and Caesarean section are frequent (Table 4.1). In these infants, breech presentation is caused by a large head or by paralytic extension of the lower limbs

TABLE 4.1. (a) Presentation and (b) mode of delivery in 130 consecutive cases of myelomeningocele.

(a)	No.	%
Vertex	106	81
(External cephalic version)	16	12
Face	1	1
Breech	23	18
—full	6	5
—frank	17	13

(b)	No.	%
Spontaneous or low forceps	85	66
Kiellands, mid cavity or ventouse	15	12
Assisted breech	16	11
Caesarean section	14	11

(Stark and Drummond, 1970). Operative delivery of a grossly malformed infant is all too common a tragedy. As a result of malpresentation, obstetric difficulty and the child's inherent vulnerability, many are in poor condition at birth or suffer some form of injury in the process (Table 4.2). The neurological disorder may be increased by damage to the brain or exposed spinal cord. In breech deliveries, there may also be damage to nerves and muscles of the lower limbs (Ráliš, 1975).

23

TABLE 4.2. Birth injury in 130 consecutive cases of myelomeningocele.

	No.	%
Cephalhaematoma	4	3
Fractures	4	3
Rupture myelomeningocele	13	10
Hyperexcitability	6	5
Apathy	11	9
Convulsions	2	2
Other	17	13

The open myelomeningocele is liable to infection during delivery and subsequently in the neonatal period from its proximity to the heavily contaminated napkin area. Infection is particularly common if the lesion has ruptured and in untreated infants colonization with staphylococci and coliform organisms is almost invariable. Suppuration of the myelomeningocele spreads readily to the subarachnoid space and leads

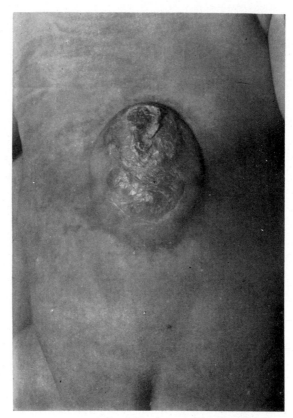

FIG. 4.1. Spontaneous epithelialization of open myelomeningocele.

to ascending meningitis and ventriculitis, the usual cause of death in untreated patients. There is, nevertheless, a striking tendency for epithelial cells to grow in over the exposed neural plate after birth, a phenomenon which explains the long-term survival of occasional untreated children. Such children are, however, usually left with an ugly, fragile and often tender swelling on the back (Fig. 4.1).

Chapter 5

Lower Limbs

The disorder of spinal cord function may be a direct result of the primary developmental anomaly. There is evidence, however, that secondary mechanisms are involved in many cases (Stark, 1972a). These include prenatal traction on the abnormally tethered spinal cord, direct pressure and longitudinal shearing forces during delivery and postnatal drying and infection of the neural plate.

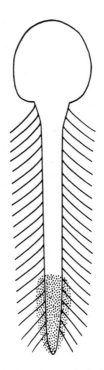

FIG. 5.1. Type I neurological lesion.

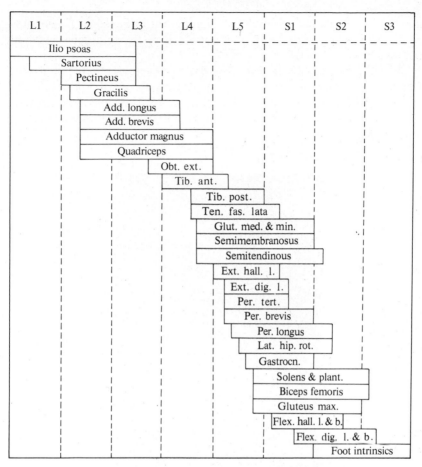

F1G. 5.2. Segmental innervation of lower limb muscles.

Patterns of Paralysis

As might be expected from the multiplicity of damaging factors at work on the spinal cord, the neurological picture in the lower limbs is not uniform in all patients. It depends on both the level and pattern of the spinal cord lesion. At birth, two main types of neurological involvement of the lower limbs can be recognized (Stark and Baker, 1967).

Type I (Fig. 5.1). Although often considered to be the typical finding in myelomeningocele, it is encountered in only one-third of patients in the neonatal period. The Type I lesion is characterized by complete loss of spinal cord function below a certain segmental level resulting in flaccid paralysis, loss of sensation and reflexes. With a knowledge of the root innervation of lower limb muscles, summarized in Fig. 5.2, the extent of cord involvement can readily be determined as the following examples will show.

The child illustrated in Fig. 5.3 has complete loss of spinal cord function below T8. Muscles innervated below this level are flaccid and there is paradoxical bulging of abdominal muscles during the expiratory phase of crying. In the absence of muscle imbalance, the lower limbs are undeformed.

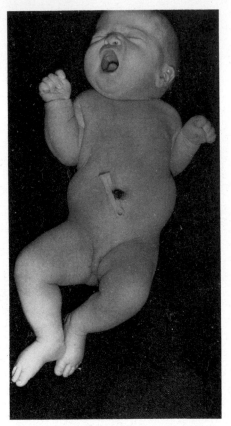

FIG. 5.3. Type I lesion: motor level T8.

Fig. 5.4 shows the typical appearance of an infant with normal function to L4 but complete paralysis below. Psoas, adductors, quadriceps and tibialis anterior (innervated from L1–4) are strong and have completely overcome their flaccid antagonists (innervated from L5 and below).

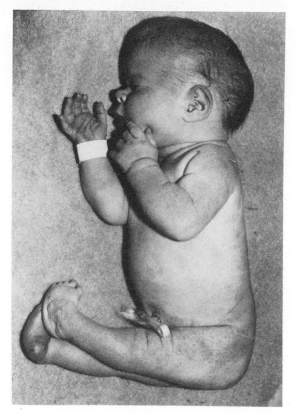

Fig. 5.4. Type I lesion: motor level L4.

If spinal cord function is spared down to L5 (Fig. 5.5), toe extensors, peronei and medial hamstrings are also active but calf muscles (S1–2) still very weak.

With normal function to S2, both dorsiflexion and plantarflexion are strong and the long toe flexors are active. There is, however, paralysis of the short toe flexors and other intrinsic muscles of the foot (S2–3). As a result, the forefoot and heel are pulled up causing the foot to break at the unsupported mid-tarsal joint (Fig. 5.6). The resultant boat-shaped or 'rocker-bottom' foot is associated with a vertical talus (Fig. 5.7).

If the lesion involves only the terminal cord segments (S4–5), there is no significant lower limb weakness but paralysis of the pelvic floor which produces the 'flat-bottomed' appearance with patulous anus illustrated in Fig. 5.8.

Type II. This pattern, found in two-thirds of infants with myelomeningo-cele, is characterized by interruption of long spinal tracts with preserva-

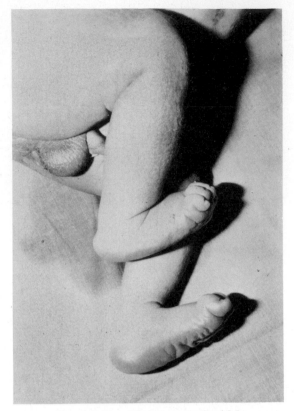

FIG. 5.5. Type I lesion: motor level L5.

tion of purely reflex activity (which may be grossly exaggerated) in isolated distal segments. Three sub-types can be recognized (Fig. 5.9).

(a) In some infants, cord function is intact down to a certain level below which there is a 'gap' manifested by flaccid paralysis, loss of sensation and reflexes. More distally, however, isolated cord function is evident from exaggerated reflex activity. For example, Fig. 5.10 shows a child with flaccid paralysis of muscles innervated from L1–5 and spastic paralysis in those supplied by S1–5 including biceps femoris, calves and toe flexors. In such infants, as a result of pelvic floor spasticity, the anus is set in a deep natal cleft (Fig. 5.11).

(b) In others, especially in the newborn period, the 'gap' in cord function is narrow, amounting virtually to a transection. There is no movement of the lower limbs when the infant is crying but a wealth of purely reflex activity, including flexion withdrawal, can be elicited by direct stimulation (Fig. 5.12).

(c) If transection of the long tracts is incomplete, the child will have a

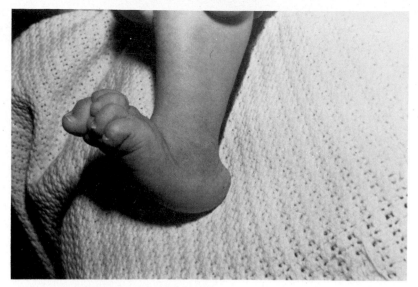

FIG. 5.6. Type I lesion: motor level S1–2.

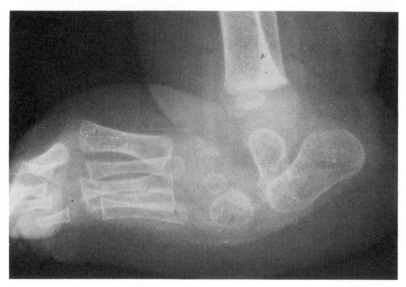

FIG. 5.7. X-ray of rocker-bottom foot.

spastic paraplegia with preservation of some voluntary movement and sensation.

In about 5 per cent of infants, notably those with a hemimyelomeningocele, while one leg is affected with a Type I or II lesion, the other is more

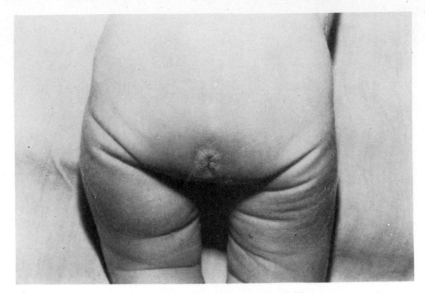

FIG. 5.8. Type I lesion: motor level S3.

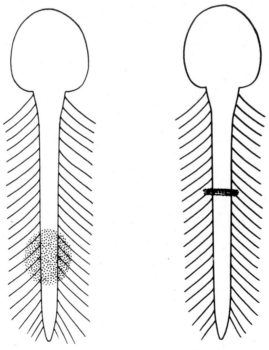

FIG. 5.9. (a and b) Type II neurological lesions. For explanation, see text.

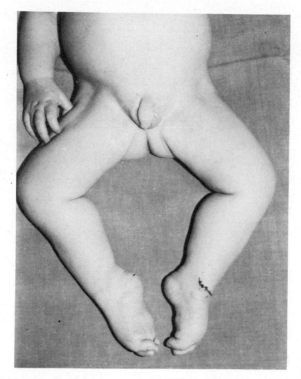

FIG. 5.10. Type IIa lesion: motor level T12; isolated cord function S1–5.

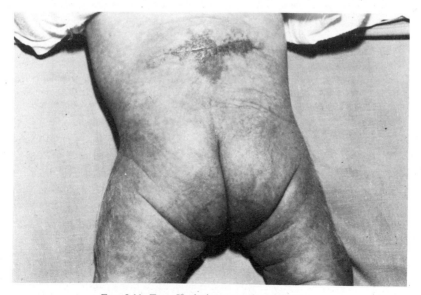

FIG. 5.11. Type IIa lesion: spastic pelvic floor.

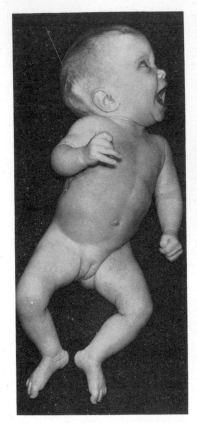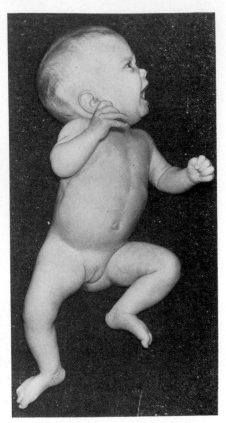

FIG. 5.12. Type IIb lesion; (a) Undeformed lower limbs at rest. (b) Flexion withdrawal reflex.

or less completely spared. Although such patients usually have normal bladder function, they are often severely disabled by the kyphoscoliosis which tends to accompany a hemimyelomeningocele (Fig. 5.13).

Isolated *nerve root lesions* are extremely rare in open myelomeningocele, which is essentially a spinal cord lesion. They may, however, occasionally occur in patients with closed myelomeningocele.

Mechanisms of Deformity

In general, as summarized in Table 5.1, muscles which displace the limb forwards are innervated from more proximal cord segments than those which move it backwards. Therefore, since agonists and antagonists do not share the same segmental innervation, cord lesions of the kind already described will frequently result in muscle imbalance. Three varieties of imbalance can be recognized:

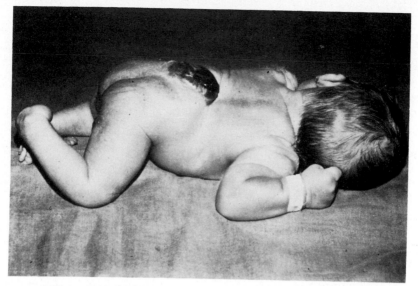

FIG. 5.13. Kyphoscoliosis associated with hemimyelomeningocele.

(a) normal muscle v. flaccid antagonist,
(b) spastic muscle v. normal antagonist, and
(c) (the most extreme) spastic muscle v. flaccid antagonist.
Muscle imbalance will cause an abnormal posture of the limb as already illustrated. It is axiomatic also that, in the growing child, it will culminate in fixed deformity. As Sharrard (1962) has clearly shown, growth of the strong, unopposed muscle is impaired while elongation of its weak antagonist is excessive.

Dislocation of the hip is an excellent example of the relationship between segmental innervation, muscle imbalance and deformity, a relationship summarized in Fig. 5.14. If the muscles around the hip are either normal or totally paralysed, there is no danger of dislocation which depends on imbalance between hip flexors and adductors (L1–3) on the one hand and gluteal extensors and abductors (L5–S2) on the

TABLE 5.1. Segmental innervation of the chief lower limb movements.

		Displacement of the Limb		
	Forwards		Backwards	
Hip	Flexion	L1–2	Extension	S1–2
Knee	Extension	L3–4	Flexion	L5–S1
Ankle	Dorsiflexion	L4–5	Plantarflexion	S1–2
Toes	Extension	L5–S1	Flexion	S2–3

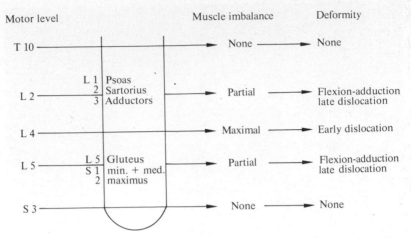

FIG. 5.14. Relationship of motor level to dislocation of the hip.

other. If imbalance is maximal, i.e. with an L4 motor level, dislocation is likely to be present at birth or to develop in the first year of life. With partial imbalance, i.e. L2 or L5 motor level, early dislocation is unlikely but increasing flexion-adduction contracture and later subluxation can be expected.

There is evidence that the important upper motor neurone lesion in Type II patients occurs around the time of birth. Deformities due to spasticity such as knee flexion and equinus contracture are, therefore, not present at birth but develop, often rapidly, in the early months of life.

While the importance of muscle imbalance cannot be exaggerated, fixed deformity can be present at birth in totally paralysed lower limbs (Fig. 5.15). In some such cases, deformity may be all that is left to show that muscle power (and imbalance) has been present in fetal life. In other cases, however, the pattern of deformity suggests that it has resulted simply from the pressure of the uterus on paralysed limbs (Stark and Drummond, 1971; Ráliš, 1974). Deformity can also develop after birth in flaccid legs which are allowed to lie constantly in one posture determined by gravity. In this way, the hips may become fixed in external rotation, the knees in flexion and the feet in equinus. Weight-bearing on totally paralysed feet will tend to force them into valgus at the subtalar joint.

Sensory Loss

Sensory loss in the trunk and lower limbs usually coincides, within a segment or two, with loss of voluntary movement. It has several important consequences.

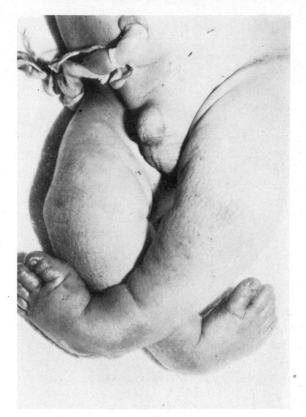

FIG. 5.15. Fixed deformities in totally paralysed lower limbs.

Aggravation of motor handicap. Development and control of normal movement depend on sensory feedback from the weight-bearing surfaces of the feet and from receptors in muscles, tendons and joints. The child with a myelomeningocele has impairment of proprioceptive sensation as well as muscular weakness. Successful achievement of walking is, therefore, considerably more difficult than for the polio victim with a comparable degree of paralysis.

Predisposition to skin breakdown. As a result of defective pain and temperature sensation, trauma may go unnoticed until there is frank ulceration of the skin. Burns and scalds occur very easily from contact with radiators or hot water bottles or from spilling of hot liquids on the skin. In the first year of life, the infant may gnaw his anaesthetic big toe to the bone, especially if varus deformity of the foot makes it unusually accessible. Later, skin breakdown may occur from pressure of ill-fitting footwear, calipers, plaster casts or the badly adjusted footrest of a wheelchair. The skin is most vulnerable over abnormal bony prominences: prolonged weight-bearing on deformed, e.g. varus feet can be disastrous. Since anaesthesia is most often present in the sacral territory, pressure sores readily occur over the lower sacrum and ischial tuberosities in the child with very limited mobility. The liability to skin breakdown is further increased by maceration from urinary incontinence and ischaemia from the vasomotor disturbance which may complicate myelomeningocele. The incidence of pressure sores has been shown to increase with age, possibly reflecting the increase in plantar pressure that normally occurs throughout childhood as body weight increases more rapidly than the weight-bearing surface of the foot (Hay and Walker, 1973). Furthermore, in spina bifida children, not only is there often a reduction in the weight-bearing surface of the foot but, as Hayes-Allen and Tring (1973) have shown, the incidence of obesity is high.

Pathological fractures. Sensory loss is an important factor also in causation of fractures of lower limb bones weakened by disuse atrophy. James (1970) reported an 18 per cent incidence in patients under his orthopaedic care, and in many, fractures were recurrent. The commonest site is the shaft of the femur which is particularly vulnerable after immobilization for hip surgery. Fractures which may occur from trivial or unrecognized trauma usually present with a hot, fusiform swelling of the limb that may suggest a diagnosis of osteomyelitis. Callus formation is often advanced before the fracture is recognized. Epiphyseal separation, chip fractures of the metaphyseal ends and subperiosteal haemorrhage are a hazard of physiotherapy and may closely mimic the radiological features of the battered baby syndrome (Edvardsen, 1972).

It might be wondered whether preservation of the sensory side of the spinal reflex arc in patients with Type II neurological patterns would provide protection against skin breakdown and pathological fractures. A recent comparison of patients with Type I and II lesions suggested that isolated reflex function conferred no such advantage (Smith *et al.*, 1973).

Chapter 6

Bladder, Bowel and Sexual Function

Bladder—Physiology and Pathophysiology

The normal bladder has two opposite and alternating functions—storage and evacuation. Balance and coordination between the two depend on control exerted by the central nervous system.

As illustrated diagramatically in Fig. 6.1, detrusor contraction and bladder sensation (fullness and desire to void) depend on parasympathetic nerves, the pelvic splanchnics, from the S2–4 segments of the spinal cord. The internal sphincter is simply a condensation of circular detrusor muscle at the bladder neck; by virtue of the radial insertion of longitudinal muscle bands it opens passively during bladder con-

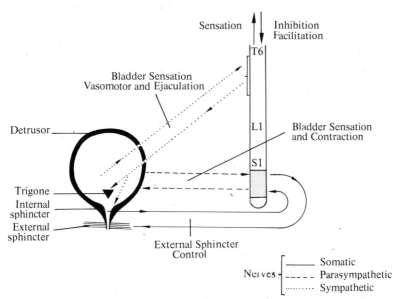

FIG. 6.1. Nerve supply of the bladder (After J. Cosbie Ross (1956) Treatment of the bladder in paraplegia. *British Journal of Urology*, **28**, 14).

traction in a manner analogous to dilatation of the uterine cervix in labour. The sympathetic nerve supply to the internal sphincter and trigone does not appear to be necessary for normal micturition (Learmonth, 1931).

The striated external sphincter, part of the pelvic diaphragm, is innervated by the somatic pudendal nerves from S2–4 which also carry afferent fibres from the posterior urethra.

In short, the 2nd to 4th sacral segments can be regarded as the spinal cord centre for bladder control. It is, in turn, regulated by the hypothalamus and cerebral cortex with which it has both afferent and efferent connections through the long spinal tracts.

Detrusor function can conveniently be studied by continuous recording of intravesical pressure through a suprapubic catheter during slow bladder filling (Sandøe et al., 1959). In the normal infant, although the tension in the bladder wall increases in a linear fashion, intravesical pressure rises only slowly during filling (Fig. 6.2). At a critical level of filling, tension receptors are stimulated and lead to reflex detrusor contraction. The intravesical pressure rises to about 40 mmHg and, as urine enters the posterior urethra, there is reflex relaxation of the external sphincter. The bladder empties with a good stream and pressure falls to the resting level. During detrusor contraction, the child shows evidence of bladder sensation. In older children and adults, reflex detrusor contractions can, of course, be inhibited for a time and, conversely, even if the bladder is not full, contraction can be initiated directly by act of will.

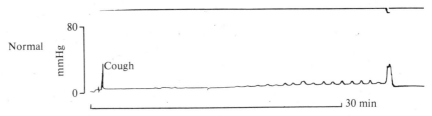

FIG. 6.2. Normal intravesical pressure recording (voiding indicated by marker above tracing).

There is a close correlation, in patients with myelomeningocele, between the neurological disorder in the lower limbs and that in the bladder (Stark, 1968, 1973a). Normal bladder activity is found only in children who have intact neurological function in at least one leg or who suffer from no more than a mild upper motor neurone lesion (Duckworth et al., 1968; Stark, 1968; Ericsson et al., 1970). In more than 90 per cent, however, spinal cord control of the bladder is defective.

Just as Type I and Type II lesions produce predominantly flaccid or spastic paralysis in the lower limbs, so, in the urinary tract, two main types of dysfunction can be recognized. These are the *inert* and *reflex* bladders which occur in approximately one-third and two-thirds of patients respectively.

Inert bladder. On pressure studies, this is characterized by a featureless tracing with no definite detrusor contractions (Fig. 6.3). There is no evidence of sensation but small volume dribbling occurs after a variable degree of filling. Manual expression is usually possible with ease. This type of bladder is associated with flaccid paralysis, sensory loss and absence of reflex activity in S2–4 territory in the lower limbs (see Chapter 11).

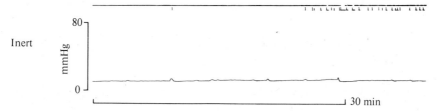

FIG. 6.3. Inert bladder: note low pressure and constant dribbling.

Reflex bladder (Fig. 6.4). Pressure recording reveals detrusor activity which is frequently strong but poorly coordinated and unaccompanied by signs of bladder sensation. Contractions may be intermittent and result in voiding of urine in a stream or they may be almost continuous with constant dribbling. The ideal 'automatic' bladder which fills without leakage and periodically empties without residue is very rare in myelomeningocele. A high intravesical pressure is often generated from failure of the external sphincter to relax during detrusor contractions (detrusor-sphincter dyssynergia). The abnormal reflex bladder is associated with either limited voluntary function or purely reflex activity in S2–4 territory in the lower limbs.

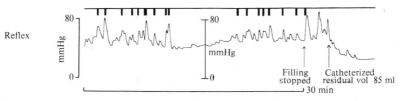

FIG. 6.4. Uninhibited reflex bladder: note high pressure and constant dribbling.

Effects of Neurogenic Bladder

With lack of spinal cord control there is a breakdown in the normal separation of the bladder's opposing functions of storage and evacuation. Evacuation during storage results in *incontinence* and storage during evacuation in *stagnation* which is a constant threat to the upper urinary tract.

Incontinence. Some degree of urinary incontinence occurs in at least 90 per cent of unselected patients with myelomeningocele. In those with inert bladders it results from a combination of sensory loss and external sphincter paralysis. In children with reflex bladders, it is due to the occurrence of detrusor contractions without warning sensation. In either group it may be due to overflow from a full bladder with outlet obstruction.

Upper urinary tract damage. The complex pathogenesis of renal failure is summarized in Fig. 6.5; the more important mechanisms will now be outlined.

    Residual urine results from failure of the detrusor to overcome the bladder outlet resistance. The inert bladder may be unable even to overcome the intrinsic elastic resistance and surface tension of the internal sphincter and posterior urethra. Residual urine is an even greater problem in the reflex bladder which may be opposed by a spastic external sphincter. As the fetus secretes urine by the end of the first trimester the

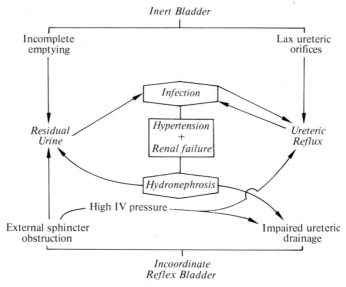

Fig. 6.5. Pathogenesis of upper urinary tract damage.

bladder may be very large by the time of birth or even rupture *in utero* (Howat, 1971).

Ureteric reflux which further increases residual urine is found in about 20 per cent of newborn infants with myelomeningocele. The incidence which increases with age is similar for inert and reflex bladders. Reflux from the former is probably due to lack of support for the ureteric orifices. From reflex bladders, the mechanism is not so much intra-vesical pressure from outlet obstruction as impairment of uretero-vesical competence by trabeculation and incoordinate detrusor activity (de Jonge *et al.,* 1959; Stark, 1973a).

Hydronephrosis was found in 15 per cent of affected newborn infants by Thomas and Hopkins (1971). Since peristalsis fails when the ureters are very dilated, it may be secondary to ureteric reflux. It can, however, develop in the absence of reflux if bladder pressure constantly exceeds the ureteric peristaltic pressure (30 mmHg) or if incoordinate detrusor activity interferes with uretero-vesical drainage.

Infection is almost inevitable if there is stagnation of the kind described above (O'Grady and Catell, 1966). In the experience of Cooper (1967) only 40 per cent of patients reached the age of 5 with uninfected urinary tracts. Stone formation is, however, surprisingly rare in children with spina bifida.

Hypertension has been reported in 50 per cent of patients with spina bifida over the age of 10 (Lorber and Lyons, 1970). Without adequate attention to the urinary tract in early childhood, a high mortality rate can, therefore, be expected from renal failure in early adult life.

Bowel—Physiology and Pathophysiology

Motility of the small bowel and proximal colon depend on para-sympathetic innervation by the vagus. Normally, the proximal colon is filled passively by ileal peristalsis. Several times a day, ingestion of food triggers a 'mass contraction' of the colon through the gastro-colic reflex, and contractions which begin in the ascending colon propel faecal material into the descending colon and rectum. In the normal infant, distension of the rectum is signalled by parasympathetic afferents to S2–4 segments of the cord from which rectal contraction is, in turn, initiated through the pelvic splanchnic (parasympathetic) nerves. In response to distension and contraction of the rectum, there is also reflex relaxation of the striated muscle of the pelvic floor—puborectalis and external anal sphincter—which has a somatic innervation from S2–4 through the pudendal nerves (Taverner and Smiddy, 1959). At the end of defaecation, the anal canal is drawn up and emptied by con-traction of the levator ani (puborectalis) and the external sphincter closes.

In the resting state, faecal continence depends on anterior angulation of the rectum by the 'pinch-cock' action of puborectalis. Leakage of flatus and liquid is prevented by tonus of the internal sphincter, the terminal circular smooth muscle of the ano-rectum, which seems to be independent of its nerve supply. In the older child, the sensation of rectal fullness is recognized and, if circumstances are inappropriate, rectal contraction is inhibited and the striated sphincter voluntarily tightened.

As a result of similarities in nerve supply, the neurogenic bowel is in many ways analogous to the bladder disturbance in myelomeningocele. As the bowel problem has been less intensively studied, it is possible to piece together only a general outline of its nature. Since the vagus nerves are seldom affected, function in the small bowel is unimpaired. Normal function of the large bowel can also be expected in children with spina bifida who develop normal bladder control.

As in the bladder, there appear to be two main types of dysfunction in the distal colon (Cuendet, 1969).

An *inert bowel* is found if there is complete loss of function in S2–4 cord, i.e. a Type I neurological lesion, and should be expected in about one-third of patients. Rectal sensation is lacking and there are no effective contractions in the descending colon and rectum. Some tone is, however, preserved in the internal sphincter (Duhamel, 1969). The striated muscle of the pelvic floor is paralysed. Loss of function in the subcutaneous external sphincter is associated with absence of the anal reflex and a characteristic 'flat-bottomed appearance' (Fig. 5.8). Of still greater importance is paralysis of the deeper striated muscle of the puborectalis sling reflected in absence of the normal ano-rectal angulation on barium enema examination described by Tsuchida *et al.* (1972) and illustrated in Fig. 6.6. In such patients, there may be a tendency to rectal prolapse.

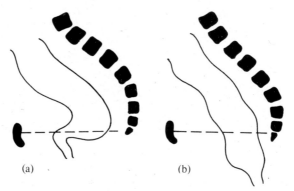

(a)   (b)

FIG. 6.6. Lateral outline of barium enema. (a) Normal infant: note anterior angulation at level of pubo-coccygeal line. (b) Pelvic floor paralysis: note sagging of ano-rectum and absence of pubo-rectalis pinchcock (After Y. Tsuchida *et al.*, 1972).

The inert bowel leads to constipation and incontinence as the anaesthetic rectum is unable to detect the rush of faeces propelled by a mass contraction and the lax anus to contain it. If the stools are very soft, continuous soiling may occur.

A *reflex bowel* is likely in the two-thirds of patients who have evidence of purely reflex activity in S2–4 segments of the spinal cord. Among this reflex activity is preservation, or even exaggeration of the anal reflex and spasticity of the pelvic floor, which results in a deep natal cleft (Fig. 5.11). Exaggeration of rectal reflex activity may also occur. Scobie *et al.,* (1970) have, for example, reported augmentation of reflex inhibition of the external sphincter on rectal distension. These patients are liable to constipation from spasticity of the pelvic floor but relatively normal defaecation may occur. Even if sensation is absent, rectal contraction may be sufficiently predictable, e.g. following meals, to permit a satisfactory degree of faecal continence. Soiling may, however, occur if there is true diarrhoea, e.g. during antibiotic therapy, or spurious diarrhoea associated with uncontrolled constipation.

Although an enormous social handicap, faecal incontinence is less constant than urinary incontinence in myelomeningocele. In the series of Scobie *et al.* (1970), although only 15 per cent had reliable urinary control, almost 50 per cent had 'perfect' bowel control.

Sexual Function

Patients suffering from neurogenic disorders of bladder and bowel are likely also to have serious difficulties in sexual relationships. Since relatively few patients with myelomeningocele have yet been followed-up into adult life, little is known of the incidence and nature of their sexual problems.

In both sexes, lack of genital sensation (S2–4) is very common and likely to interfere seriously with sexual activity although libido may be normal.

With Type I lesions involving S2–4 spinal cord, *males* are unlikely to be capable of either penile erection or ejaculation. With preservation of reflex function in S2–4, reflex erections can be expected but efficient ejaculation improbable. Their unhappy predicament was aptly described by Segalas (1844) as one of 'erections without desires which are sometimes followed by desires without erections'.

The spinal cord lesion is likely to interfere rather less with the more passive coital role of the *female*. More than a century ago, Sir James Young Simpson described successful pregnancy, labour and delivery in a paraplegic woman, a possibility confirmed by more recent reports of patients with myelomeningoceles.

Sexual adjustment in these patients is likely to be further prejudiced by incontinence and physical handicap in many cases.

It is only recently that serious attention has been directed to sexual dysfunction in spina bifida (Scott *et al.*, 1975). Much more remains to be learned not only about the physical problems of coitus but about the effect of genital anaesthesia on psychosexual development in childhood and adolescence.

Chapter 7

Associated Malformations

Like other misfortunes, congenital malformations seldom come singly. Children with myelomeningoceles have a particularly high incidence of associated anomalies even if we exclude abnormalities such as 'talipes' and hydronephrosis which are simply effects of the primary lesion of the spinal cord. Table 7.1 shows the incidence of associated anomalies in a series of 200 consecutive infants with myelomeningocele studied in the newborn period. The more important conditions will be considered in more detail.

TABLE 7.1. Associated malformations detected in newborn period in 200 consecutive infants with myelomeningocele.

Hydrocephalus	95%	(Routine AVG)
Lacunar skull	88%	(Routine skull x-ray)
Abnormal ribs	27%	(Routine chest x-ray)
Kyphosis	25% ⎫	⎰Localized Vert. Anom. 18%
Scoliosis	22% ⎭	⎱Mult. Vert. Anom. 17%
Mongoloid features	7%	
Odd features	7%	
Single tr. palmar crease	3·5%	
Genital anomalies	3·5%	(Hypospadias, undes. testes, etc.)
Ectopic/imperforate anus	1·5%	
Miscellaneous	8%	(PDA, accessory auricles, haemangiomata, Klippel-Feil, sacral agenesis etc.)

Hydrocephalus

Apart from the occasional child with a closed sacral lesion, virtually all patients with myelomeningocele have some degree of hydrocephalus. In the milder cases, however, it is detectable only by routine ventriculography and in approximately one-third it becomes arrested at an early stage without surgical treatment.

47

In patients with myelomeningocele, hydrocephalus is almost invariably associated with the Arnold-Chiari malformation which, despite its name, was first described by Cleland (1883). In this malformation there is herniation of the brainstem and cerebullar vermis through the foramen magnum so that the fourth ventricle opens into the cervical spinal canal. The cerebellum is small, deformed and depleted of Purkinjé cells: lateral compression of the midbrain results in distortion, buckling and narrowing of the aqueduct (Variend and Emery, 1973; Emery, 1974).

The cause of the Arnold-Chiari malformation has long been controversial. Initially it was though to be an effect of hydrocephalus (Chiari, 1891) but has more recently also been recognized as a cause. Penfield and Coburn (1938) attributed it to downward traction of the brainstem resulting from abnormal fixation of the spinal cord by the myelomeningocele. Barry et al. (1957) found, however, that the angulation of nerve roots was not consistent with the traction theory and favoured 'encephalo-cranial disproportion' as a cause, i.e. foramen magnum coning from overgrowth of nerve tissue which has often been observed in both brain and spinal cord of spina bifida patients. For a critical review of the pathogenesis of the brainstem malformation, the reader is referred to Caviness (1976).

No less complex than its origin are the ways in which the Arnold-Chiari malformation causes hydrocephalus. It could theoretically obstruct the flow of cerebrospinal fluid at three main sites; foramen magnum, fourth ventricale and aqueduct of Sylvius. Plugging of the foramen magnum by the prolapsed cerebellar tonsils would result in communicating hydrocephalus, i.e. hydrocephalus in which there is free flow between the ventricular system and the spinal theca but obstruction in the subarachnoid space which prevents cerebrospinal fluid reaching its main absorption site in the arachnoid villi. Internal hydrocephalus in which cerebrospinal fluid is unable to escape from the ventricular system would be expected from obstruction of the outlet foramina of the 4th ventricle by the closely applied cerebellar tonsils or from the secondary aqueduct obstruction. The relative importance of obstruction at these sites varies in individual children so that hydrocephalus associated with myelomeningocele may be predominantly communicating or internal in type. In practice, neuroradiological studies have shown that it is communicating in one-third and internal in two-thirds of patients (Milhorat, 1972; Drummond and Donaldson, 1974).

Although ventricular dilatation is usually present at birth the affected infant need not have a large head; only 25 per cent of newborns with myelomeningocele have an occipito-frontal circumference above the 90th centile. Rapid head enlargement and increase in intracranial pressure tend to occur after birth and repair of the myelomeningocele. Postnatal progression of hydrocephalus was formerly attributed to removal by back closure of a cerebrospinal fluid absorption site. More recently, Wealthall (1973) has suggested that what is removed with the myelomeningocele sac is rather a mechanism for damping sharp pressure rises transmitted to the spinal theca. Williams (1971) has advanced a theory which, even if it does not completely explain the development of the Arnold-Chiari malformation, could account for postnatal deterioration. He has shown that on crying and straining, which are essentially postnatal habits, the pressure rise in the lumbar theca precedes that in the basal cisterns establishing a pressure gradient which drives cerebrospinal fluid upwards past the Arnold-Chiari malformation; when the baby relaxes and pressure falls it does so earlier in the lumbar theca reversing the pressure gradient and impacting the hind brain more firmly in the foramen magnum. This valvular mechanism which would operate with or without operation on the myelomeningocele could increase both the Arnold-Chiari malformation and the consequent aqueduct compression.

The most obvious pathological effects of hydrocephalus are dilatation of the ventricular system proximal to the obstruction, breakdown of the septum pellucidum and thinning of the cerebral mantle, which is normally 35 mm at birth (Fig. 7.1). Histologically, there is disruption of the ependymal lining of the ventricles with cerebrospinal fluid oedema and destruction of nerve fibres and myelin in the white matter of the cerebral hemispheres. Considerable ventricular dilatation may take place without significant cell loss from the cortical grey matter (Weller *et al.*, 1969; Rubin *et al.*, 1972).

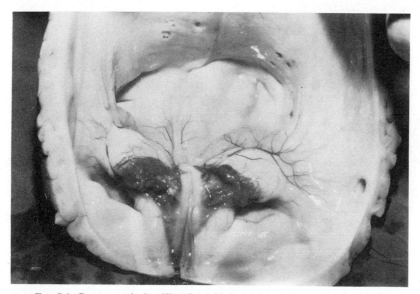

FIG. 7.1. Gross ventricular dilatation with breakdown of septum pellucidum.

Abnormally rapid head growth may be the outstanding or only clinical feature in early infancy when cranial bones are easily separated. While some normal infants have a wide anterior fontanelle and sagittal suture in the newborn period, marked separation of the lambdoidal suture and prominence of the frontal region are particularly suggestive of hydro-cephalus. Even if it is not particularly large the hydrocephalic head feels softer than normal.

If the hydrocephalus is not arrested spontaneously or by treatment, after a period of days, weeks or months, the limits of compliance of the infant's head are reached and signs of raised intracranial pressure develop (Fig. 7.2). This stage is reached particularly rapidly in infants with the least ventricular enlargement. The child's behaviour is characterized by vomiting and irritability. On examination, the anterior fontanelle is tense and bulging and percussion of the skull may yield a dull 'crackpot' sound. The scalp has a shiny appearance and there is prominence of superficial veins due to interference with intracranial venous drainage.

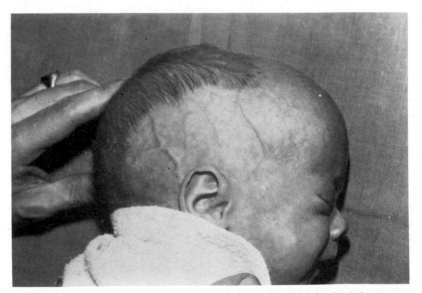

Fig. 7.2. Clinical features of raised intracranial pressure in infancy.
(a) Prominent scalp veins.

The earliest neurological sign of raised pressure is commonly impaired upward conjugate deviation of the eyes resulting in the well-known 'sunset' sign. The underlying lesion in the tectum of the midbrain has been ascribed to pressure on it from tentorial herniation of the supra-pineal recess of the 3rd ventricle (Shillat et al., 1973). In long-standing hydrocephalus the sunset sign is accentuated by depression of the

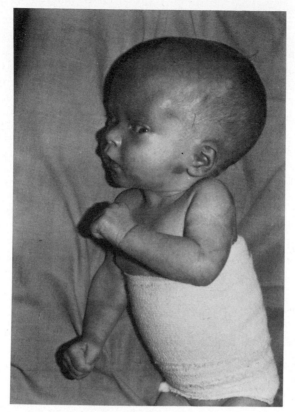

FIG. 7.2. Clinical features of raised intracranial pressure in infancy.
(b) Extensor hypertonus with strong ATNR.

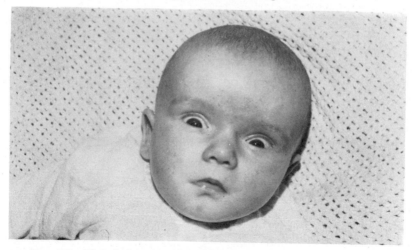

FIG. 7.2. Clinical features of raised intracranial pressure in infancy.
(c) Sunset sign.

orbital roofs. If pressure is unrelieved, convergent strabismus due to a lesion of the vulnerable 6th nerve often develops and may be accompanied by retinal venous congestion and papilloedema. With increasing brainstem compression, extensor hypertonus appears with exaggeration of asymmetrical tonic neck reflex, head retraction and opisthotonus. Finally, with decerebration, there is breakdown of homeostasis and death ensues.

Longer term effects of hydrocephalus on cerebral function will be considered in Chapter 8.

Malformations of the Axial Skeleton

In addition to separation of sutures and shallowness of the posterior cranial fossa associated with hydrocephalus and the Arnold-Chiari malformation, the so-called *lacunar skull* is very common (Fig. 7.3). The skull is thin and there are roughly circular areas in which ossification is particularly defective. The configuration is not that of cortical impression, is unrelated to raised intracranial pressure and disappears within the first few months of life. It is almost always associated with

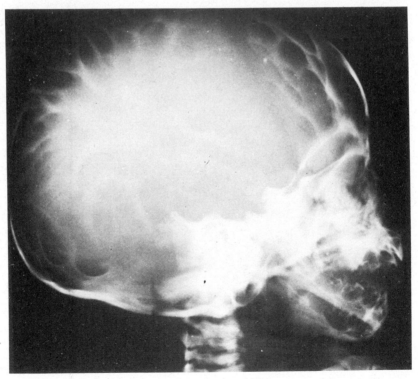

FIG. 7.3. Lacunar skull.

myelomeningocele and may be a useful radiological sign of fetal abnormality in late pregnancy.

In addition to the vertebral arch defect at the site of the myelomeningocele almost 50 per cent of affected infants have significant and commonly disabling spinal deformity.

Kyphosis occurs most frequently in those with extensive thoracolumbar lesions in whom it may be associated with multiple vertebral anomalies (Fig. 7.4). In such cases, wide separation and eversion of the pedicles and laminae of bifid vertebrae leads to lateral and anterior displacement of erector spinae muscles which lose their extensor function and, in conjunction with active psoas muscles and diaphragm, act like a bowstring to increase the deformity (Drennan, 1970). The angle of the kyphotic deformity is commonly less than 90°. Whatever the neurological level, walking, standing and even comfortable sitting are prejudiced, orthopaedic and urinary diversion appliances difficult to fit when the costal margin is virtually resting on the iliac crest and skin breakdown over the bony prominence a chronic problem.

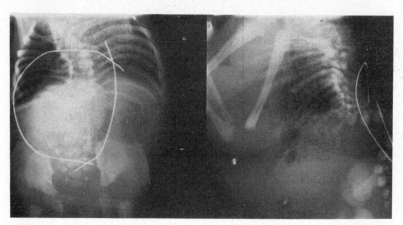

FIG. 7.4. X-ray of congenital kyphosis with multiple vertebral anomalies: wire markers outline myelomeningocele.

Scoliosis is related to anomalous vertebral development such as hemivertebrae which may be associated with fusion of the transverse processes of adjacent vertebrae or of ribs (Fig. 7.5). Such anomalies may be present at the level of the myelomeningocele, e.g. in hemimyelomeningocele, or at a higher level. When it occurs in the thoracic or thoracolumbar regions, scoliosis is usually accompanied by an element of kyphosis, whereas in the lumbosacral spine there is a tendency to lordo-scoliosis. Although not invariable, progressive deterioration commonly occurs as

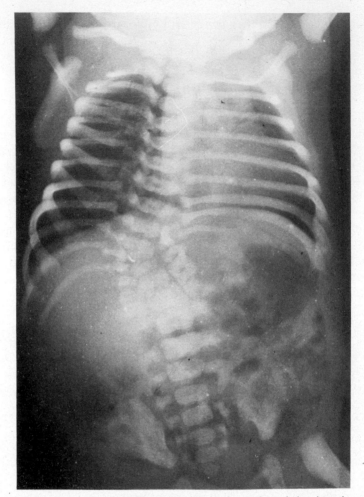

FIG. 7.5. X-ray of congenital scoliosis showing lower thoracic hemivertebrae and absence of ribs on left.

gravity accentuates the spinal curvature to produce wedging of the growing vertebrae (Winter *et al.*, 1968). Scoliosis increases the functional impact of lower limb deformity by causing a pelvic tilt and may lead to a severe and ugly deformity of the chest.

Scoliosis can, of course, also be caused by or aggravated by asymmetrical paralysis of the trunk or lower limbs.

Lordosis of the lumbar spine appears to be due to a combination of defective posterior vertebral elements and fixed flexion of the hips from unopposed psoas activity. It is seldom present at birth but tends to develop in later childhood and to increase with the puberty growth spurt.

Thoracic Malformation

Apart from deformity secondary to kyphosis or scoliosis, true developmental anomalies of the thoracic spine are very common. These include supernumerary, absent, bifid or fused ribs which are, however, usually of little functional importance and are detected only on radiological examination.

Genitourinary anomalies

Abnormalities of the external genitalia, e.g. hypospadias, cryptorchidism, occur with increased frequency in infants with myelomeningocele. Although the major pathological changes in the urinary tract described in Chapter 6 result from the neurogenic bladder, true developmental anomalies are encountered in 10–20 per cent of cases coming to autopsy (Roberts, 1961; Wilcock and Emery, 1970). Lesions such as horseshoe, pelvic or cystic kidneys are pre-eminent but escape detection on clinical examination.

Other malformations

A mongoloid facial appearance with slanting eyes and epicanthic folds is not uncommon in the newborn and may be arresting enough to prompt chromosome study; in such patients, however, the chromosomes are normal and the facial appearance becomes more normal as time goes by. As noted in Table 7.1, a wide variety of other malformations may be detected on clinical examination, the more important of which are imperforate anus and congenital heart disease. The individual incidence of such malformations is, however, no more than 1 per cent.

Rarely myelomeningocele occurs as one of a constellation of serious anomalies in the 18-trisomy syndrome (Passarge *et al.*, 1966).

Lister, 1971; de Lange, 1974). When confronted with ethical problems such as those of spina bifida, the individual doctor can do no more than seek to resolve them in a way which is acceptable to his own conscience, in accord with the feelings of society and, above all, in the best interests of his patient. In this situation, different opinions and shades of opinion are inevitable even among the best informed members of the profession and of the community. There is no single, simple, right solution and per-haps the only view that can be absolutely wrong is the dogmatic assertion that there is. While respecting contrary views, the author has found that the following considerations make the practice of selective treatment compatible with relative peace of mind.

The problem of selection for treatment is by no means peculiar to myelomeningocele. Medical progress in the last 20 years, including developments in assisted ventilation, haemodialysis and organ transplant-ation have made it theoretically possible to prolong survival of the most grossly malformed infants such as anencephalic and cyclopean monsters who would otherwise die soon after birth. Unless it is argued that doctors are morally obliged to deploy every available therapeutic measure in every case to prolong life, a view which is not even held in the Vatican (Villot, 1970), the real point at issue is where we should draw the line. The standpoint of the doctor who considers that, on the evidence of results of present treatment, the line should be drawn through myelomeningo-cele is, in moral terms, no different from those who advocate routine early closure but shrink from resuscitation of infants with anencephaly.

Selection for treatment implies not that the unselected child should be killed or even encouraged to die but that he should be *allowed* to die in peace and with the least possible suffering. Since it is operation which changes the natural history of myelomeningocele, it is the decision to operate which requires justification rather than the decision to withhold it.

Finally, priorities in medicine are inescapable. Optimal management of children with myelomeningocele makes heavy demands on medical, surgical, social and educational resources, all of which are and always will be limited. Large-scale practice of routine early operation would not only impinge on the treatment of children with other congenital mal-formations but would sooner or later prejudice optimal management of spina bifida patients with good prospects of independence. Selective treatment, at best an unhappy compromise, is suggested not as a final solution but only as an acceptable approach to management in countries such as the U.K. at the present time. Even such a limited operation policy may be unjustifiable in developing countries where countless children die from preventable or treatable infective and nutritional disorders and in which there are no facilities for habilitation of the handicapped child. In the future also, when prevention is a reality, selection for treatment will become irrelevant.

Chapter 10

Organization of Treatment

Myelomeningocele with associated hydrocephalus is a classical example of the increasing problem of multiple handicaps and their management. No single doctor can cope adequately with all the clinical problems which may arise in the fields of paediatrics, neurology, neurosurgery, urology, orthopaedics, plastic surgery and ophthalmology. Other, and no less serious problems require nursing, social work, therapy, psychology and other disciplines for their solution. The dilemma which arises is one of ensuring specialized skills for all the child's needs without causing confusion and exhaustion from multiple clinic attendances and without jeopardizing continuity of care. Two developments have helped to resolve the dilemma.

Centralization of Hospital Treatment

Regional treatment centres have evolved in most of the paediatric teaching hospitals and in general hospitals in the larger centres of population. A comprehensive assessment and treatment service for spina bifida can be justified in hospitals serving a population of half a million to one million which can expect to admit 25–50 new patients per annum in the U.K. Although it is not always possible to assemble all the necessary specialist facilities in a single hospital, the need to admit a child to several hospitals or even several units within one hospital makes coordination of care more difficult. In different centres, centralization of hospital care has been achieved in different ways. In the Royal Hospital for Sick Children, Edinburgh, for example, the paediatric neurology unit is recognized as the child's base. Whatever the clinical problem, he is, as far as possible, admitted to the same ward where senior nursing staff have a special interest and experience in all aspects of spina bifida. The ward sister becomes a familiar figure to child and parents who come to recognize her as a valuable source of practical advice and support. The child is seen in the unit by the various medical and surgical specialists in the team and, if operation is required, pre- and post-operative care are given in the same unit. As paediatric surgery has traditionally been well developed in Scotland, surgical management is simplified by the paediatric surgeon accepting responsibility for back closure, cerebrospinal fluid shunts and urological procedures. A paediatric neurosurgeon joins ward rounds and deals with the more complex problems in his field. In-patient orthopaedic management is in a neighbouring orthopaedic hospital.

In other centres, tradition or convenience have dictated centralization of in-patient treatment in the paediatric surgical or neurosurgical unit. The nature of the unit involved is less important than avoidance of admission to many different units, particularly those with adult orientation.

Combined Clinics

Even if in-patient care cannot be concentrated in a single unit or hospital, out-patient follow-up can, with great advantage, be in a combined spina bifida clinic. As a result of local circumstances and case-load, different patterns of combined clinic have emerged.

In the Royal Hospital for Sick Children, Edinburgh, the child is reviewed (generally at intervals of 4–6 months) simultaneously in a large room by a paediatrician with a special interest in neurology, a paediatric surgeon and orthopaedic surgeon. The neurological ward sister, physiotherapist, occupational therapist and medical social worker are also in attendance. After each specialist has examined the child, the next stage in management is discussed by the group and with the parents. In this way each member of the team is clearly aware of his colleagues' plans for the patient and a concerted programme of management is possible. The optimal timing of hip surgery in relation to operation on the urinary tract can be discussed: the orthopaedic surgeon can ensure that a urinary diversion stoma is kept well away from future braces, and other potentially troublesome problems can be resolved with ease. The joint clinic also provides a meeting place for parents and an opportunity for group discussion with social worker or therapists. A joint clinic along these lines is feasible only if numbers are relatively small and certainly no more than 10 patients are attending. While the combined clinic is the focal point of out-patient management, the child with a predominantly medical problem such as urinary tract infection may be seen in the interim by the paediatrician alone, and may attend the orthopaedic clinic in the early post-operative period or for modification of calipers.

In Oxford, the clinic is arranged differently from the 'circus' just described. The child stays in a cubicle and is visited by each specialist in turn. At the end of the clinic members of the medical team meet to discuss each child and then convey their collective advice to parents (Hide and Semple, 1970).

In Sheffield, where patients are more numerous, yet another arrangement has been adopted. Each specialist occupies a separate room and patients are directed from one to another as necessary. In this way every child need not see every doctor at each clinic visit. As in other centres, however, members of the team can discuss patients with one another.

In Sydney, instead of organizing a combined clinic, a medical 'co-ordinator' attends each specialty clinic with the child and acts as a link between them (Field, 1972).

Although the combined clinic facilitates communication between members of the team, it is difficult for a committee to establish the rapport which is essential for communication with parents. A corollary of the team approach is, therefore, the need for a coordinator who can listen to the parents' problems and convey to them the advice of the team. In many centres the paediatrician has emerged as coordinator; at times, however, when orthopaedic or urinary tract problems are pre-eminent the role of coordinator may be fulfilled by the orthopaedic or paediatric surgeon.

Well-coordinated specialist services in a regional centre are, however, only one facet of management of the child with spina bifida and his family. The child's real life may be lived many miles away and it is there that the impact of his handicap on everyday activities, family life and education will be felt. No less important is the need for communication with the family doctor, school health service, community nurses, social workers and therapists. By involving these workers who are strategically placed, many of the child's needs can be met in his own community.

Although communication from the hospital is traditionally by letter, there is a case also for more direct contacts with those responsible for the child's care in the community. Visits by hospital nurses, social workers and therapists to meet their counterparts have proved invaluable. Medical members of the team, especially the paediatrician, can also make rewarding forays into the community. By holding follow-up clinics for handicapped children in district hospitals, assessment centres or even the larger health centres and by visiting special schools for physically handicapped children, closer liaison can be achieved with family doctors and school doctors. As a result of such visits, both parents and children come to see their local doctors, nurses and therapists as an extension of the hospital team they have come to trust. More of the child's problems can be overcome locally and the frequency of visits to the regional combined clinic reduced.

Although he has a potentially outstanding role in management, the family doctor is often by-passed as a result of the initial direct referral from the maternity hospital to the paediatric unit, the necessity of specialized hospital follow-up and the apparent complexity of the problems which leads parents to turn so often to the hospital for help.

Involvement of family doctors in the care of handicapped children is likely to increase with the emergence, in the larger group practices and health centres, of a general practitioner with a special interest and possibly hospital attachment in paediatrics, along the lines of the Livingston New Town experiment (Stark *et al.*, 1975).

Chapter 11

Referral and Assessment

Action in the Obstetric Unit

Every infant with a myelomeningocele deserves comprehensive assessment as soon as possible after birth and should be referred to the nearest specialized unit. If a policy of selective operation is favoured it is particularly important that the decision to operate or not to operate should be taken by an experienced team with all the facts of the case available. Selection in the obstetric unit by staff with limited experience of spina bifida is fraught with danger: some of the worst-looking myelomeningoceles – large pedunculated sacs which may have ruptured during delivery – carry the most favourable prognosis. As a general rule, the infant should be retained in the obstetric unit only if his general condition is so poor that he is unlikely to survive more than a few hours.

It is essential, therefore, that general practitioners and maternity hospital staff should know the location of the nearest spina bifida unit and the procedure for transfer. Early notification by telephone is usually appreciated. Pending transfer, the baby should be nursed in an incubator, prone or on his side, with the myelomeningocele protected by a pad of sterile gauze moistened in normal saline solution. Dry dressings which can adhere to the lesion and greasy preparations such as tulle gras should be avoided as their removal may cause further damage to the exposed neural plate.

Unless the child is transferred in a portable incubator, he may be unfit for either reliable neurological assessment or early surgical treatment on arrival. In the event of an affected child being born at home, the time taken for the ambulance to collect a ready-warmed, portable incubator from the obstetric unit is well spent.

Details of the birth history should be sent with the nurse who accompanies the child. It is customary also to send a signed operation consent form; its value is, however, limited unless the parents have clearly understood the nature of the lesion and of the surgical treatment which may be required.

71

When confronted by an overwhelming crisis, human beings, like threatened herring gulls, tend to indulge in displacement activities. Every major accident generates countless cups of tea. Similarly, in the maternity hospital, nurses and doctors tend to busy themselves with the practical arrangements for the infant's transfer rather than deal with the equally urgent emotional plight of the mother.

As soon as her baby is born, every mother expects to be told its sex and that it is normal. Immediate removal of the baby, an awful silence or whispered exchanges between attendants spell alarm. Twenty-five per cent of mothers in one study knew from the reaction of staff that their babies were abnormal before they were told (Woodburn, 1974). Evasiveness at this stage can only heighten the mother's anxiety. In the larger maternity units, a paediatrician should be available to give the first information to both parents. Not infrequently, however, it falls to a nurse or midwife to break the unwelcome news (Walker *et al.,* 1971; Freeston, 1971). Fortunately, this unenviable situation is rare in any nurse's career; unfortunately, few are prepared for it by training or experience. Unless she is too heavily sedated to understand, in which case the·problem is less urgent, the mother should be gently told that her baby has an abnormality of its back and that a doctor will talk to her about it as soon as possible. As her words may be imprinted for ever on the mother's memory, the nurse should not minimize the child's defect nor dispel all hope. Comments such as, 'it's just a little gap in the skin' or, at the other extreme, 'it's better if such babies do not live' may later be very difficult to erase and may prejudice acceptance of the child. In these critical early minutes, the mother should be allowed to see and hold her baby in her arms.

Before the child is transferred, a doctor should outline the nature of the child's condition to both parents. The important message which must now be put across is that the child has a serious spinal abnormality which is usually associated with weakness of the legs and bladder; that, in some cases, a great deal can be done to help the child although complete recovery cannot be promised; that thorough early assessment is necessary to determine whether their baby can benefit from treatment. No less important is reassurance that every stage of management will be discussed with them and their inevitable questions answered with honesty. As many parents have never heard of spina bifida before, simple language must be used and the main facts repeated. The possibility of early death may be conveyed in such terms as, 'of course, even if all goes well, it will be some days before he is out of the woods'. At this juncture, it is probably unwise to become involved in detailed description of long-term problems which may never arise. Although genetic counselling must come later, the parents should be reassured that nothing they (or anyone else) did, or did not do, during the pregnancy could have caused the child's condition.

These observations are intended only as a guide to what parents should be told at the outset. Individual doctors will develop their own approach to the problem. Exactly what is said and how it is said will also be determined by the emotional state and intelligence of parents. In retrospect, however, most parents agree that 'they should tell you the worst but give you some hope' (Woodburn, 1974).

After transfer of the infant, accompanied if possible by the father, the mother is likely to be left in the maternity unit with feelings of helplessness, bewilderment and isolation. She should obviously be discharged home as soon as her own condition allows. In the meantime, however, she should not be nursed in an ordinary post-natal ward especially if babies are 'roomed-in' with their mothers. She requires privacy to express her emotions which may include guilt, inadequacy and despair. She also needs a sympathetic ear. Contact with a medical social worker is invaluable at this stage; not only can support be given but her understanding of the child's condition can be assessed and groundless fears allayed. She must be given reliable information about her baby's progress. Telephone messages can be supplemented by a visit from the medical social worker from the specialist unit who will, of course, be fully appraised of the child's condition. The family doctor can also provide both support and information in the early days. It is essential, therefore, that he be informed as soon as possible after the child's birth, and kept in touch with developments in the children's hospital.

Neonatal Assessment

Neonatal assessment of the infant with a myelomeningocele has three main objectives: to provide a basis for selection, a guide to early therapeutic needs and a base-line for later reassessment. It comprises history-taking, clinical examination and special investigation (Stark, 1971).

HISTORY
A summary of the birth history should be provided by the referring obstetric unit. The family and social history can be obtained from the father if, as recommended, he accompanies the child to the paediatric unit. Otherwise, details may be obtained from the family doctor whose personal observations may be very valuable.

CLINICAL EXAMINATION
There are several essential requirements for adequate clinical examination;
   1. an infant who is warm (temp. $>35°C$) and active but not recently fed,

2. knowledge of the segmental innervation (motor and sensory) of the lower limbs, and
3. familiarity with the various neurological patterns which may be encountered (see Chapter 5).

During examination, care must be taken to avoid direct pressure on the myelomeningocele and to prevent chilling of the infant; these are not only damaging but may invalidate neurological assessment. The examination which will be outlined can be carried out without removing the child from the incubator.

General Examination

Attention is first directed to the infant's general condition as measured by colour, temperature, respiration and level of activity. A brief but systematic examination is essential to identify associated malformations. The maximum occipitofrontal circumference should be measured and recorded on a percentile chart along with weight and length.* An OFC above the 90th percentile is suggestive of severe hydrocephalus: in Lorber's (1961) series the cerebral mantle was less than 25 mm in every such case. Hydrocephalus may, however, be equally severe in the majority of infants whose head circumference is normal at birth. Separation of the sutures, especially the lambdoidal is, therefore, a more reliable sign of hydrocephalus at birth than head size. The signs of raised intracranial pressure described in Chapter 7 are seldom striking in the first 24 hours of life.

Spinal lesion. The type of spinal lesion is first confirmed. There is no difficulty in recognizing an open myelomeningocele; occasionally, however, differentiation between a closed myelomeningocele, a simple meningocele and a lipoma (see Chapter 20) may be impossible without surgical exploration. Intact skin cover suggests a meningocele or lipoma; a narrow base and easy transillumination favour the former. Cerebrospinal fluid will usually be seen leaking on to the neural plate from the central canal at the upper end of an open myelomeningocele. Of greater significance, however, is leakage through a tear in the membranous part of the lesion which predisposes to meningitis.

Cranial nerves and upper limbs. The cranial nerves are briefly checked. For the most part this can be done by observing facial, palatal, tongue and eye movements as other aspects of the examination proceed. In the rare case of a cervicothoracic myelomeningocele, detailed examination of motor, sensory and reflex function is necessary along the lines indicated below for evaluation of the lower limbs. Otherwise, it is necessary at

* Prepared by Gairdner and Pearson, published in *Archives of Disease in Children* (1971) and obtainable from Messrs. Creasey, Bull Plain, Hertford.

this stage only to note any asymmetry of tone, posture and movement when the child is crying and when the Moro reflex is elicited.

Lower limbs. If the baby is quiet, the opportunity should be taken to carry out *sensory testing* first. If, however, he is so lethargic that even stimulation of the upper limbs evokes little or no response, testing is worthless and should be postponed. The first aim is to determine the lowest segmental level of normal sensation. Starting in the lowest sacral territory, i.e. the perianal region, the skin is stimulated with a sterile needle over the posterior aspect of the buttocks, thighs and legs and then upward over successive dermatomes of the anterior surface and on to the abdomen (Fig. 11.1). All the while, the baby is watched

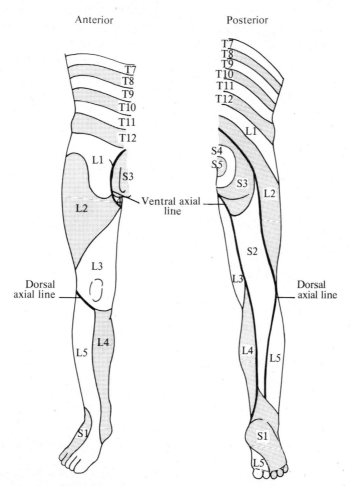

FIG. 11.1. Sensory dermatomes of the lower limbs.

closely for a facial grimace, a cry or a Moro response which indicate that sensation has reached cerebral level.

After sensory testing, the infant will usually be angry, crying and active – the ideal state for *testing of motor function*. If he is too quiet, the child may need to be goaded into activity by a flick, or other stimulation of the upper limbs. Assessment of motor function depends on the fact that the hungry, crying baby normally shows active movement of every muscle: if active arm movements are present, there should be equally strong movement in the lower limbs. Initially, 'voluntary' movement is assessed, i.e. movement which occurs synchronously with upper limb movement and crying and not only in response to direct lower limb stimulation. By appropriate positioning, each muscle can be made to operate with gravity eliminated or against gravity, e.g. with the baby carefully supported in supine, quadriceps is forced to act against gravity whereas in the lateral position it acts with gravity eliminated. If gravity can be overcome, the strength of contraction can be assessed by palpation. In this way it is possible to determine not only the presence or absence of voluntary movement but to grade its power. Although difficult to apply to certain muscles, e.g. glutei and foot intrinsics, the Medical Research Council scale, summarized in Table 11.1, has proved useful and such grading correlates well with more sophisticated electromyographic assessment (Stark and Drummond, 1972). If the scores are noted on a chart with muscles listed in descending order of segmental innervation, the voluntary motor level readily becomes apparent (Table 11.2).

TABLE 11.1. Clinical grading of muscle power. (MRC, 1943)

Grade	Description
0	No contraction
1	Flicker of contraction
2	Active movement with gravity eliminated
3	Active movement against gravity
4	Active movement against gravity and resistance
5	Normal power

After delineation of motor and sensory levels, the extent of *isolated cord function* should be explored. Lower limb territory distal to the sensory level is stimulated directly, e.g. with a straightened paper clip, and the response noted in muscles which are not under 'voluntary' control. The knee jerk (L3–4) and ankle jerk (S1–2) are also tested. On the chart, muscles showing purely reflex activity are indicated by the letter 'R'.

The neurological findings are useful in predicting increasing deformity due to muscle imbalance. For example, the child found to have a

TABLE 11.2. Neurological examination chart.

Date and Age		R	L	R	L	R	L	R	L	R	L	R	L	R	L
T	8–10 Upper abdo.														
	11–12 Lower abdo.														
L	2 Psoas														
	3–4 Adductors														
	3–4 Quadriceps														
	4 Tib. ant.														
L–S	5–1 Hamstr. med.														
	5–1 Abductors														
	5–1 Long. Ext.														
	5–1 Peronei														
S	1–2 Calf														
	1–2 Hamstr. lat.														
	1–2 Glut. max.														
	1–2 Flex. hal. long														
	1–2 Flex. dig. long														
	2–3 Intrinsics														
Reflexes															
Abdominal															
Cremasteric															
Knee															
Ankle															
Lat. hamstring															
Crossed Ext.															
Flexion withdrawal															
Motor Level															
'Voluntary'															
Isol. Cord															
Sensory Level															
Central															
Isol. Cord															

voluntary motor level of L2–3 is liable to progressive flexion-adduction contracture and later dislocation of the hip from unopposed action of psoas and adductor muscles. In the child with isolated function in S1–3 cord, knee flexion and equinus deformities can be anticipated due to spasticity of hamstring and calf muscles.

Fixed deformity already present at birth must, however, also be noted and measured, preferably by the orthopaedic member of the assessment team.

Bladder. As noted in Chapter 6 there is a close correlation between lower limb function in S2–4 territory and bladder function. The nature of this

TABLE 11.3. Correlation of lower limb function in S2–4 territory and nature of bladder activity. (Stark, 1969)

S2–4 Function in lower limbs	Bladder Activity		
	Normal	Incoordinate Reflex	Inert
Normal	+	−	−
Normal one side	+	−	−
Normal ex. mild U.M.N. lesion	+	−	−
Incomplete	−	+	−
Reflex only	−	+	−
Absent	−	−	+

association is summarized in Table 11.3 and the most useful measures of S2–4 function noted in Fig. 11.2. It should be noted that in assessing foot intrinsic muscles the most reliable sign is the presence of toe flexion at the metatarso-phalangeal joints, in the absence of which clawing of the toes is likely to be found. The toe stretch reflex (S2–3) is elicited by flicking the toes into extension. If it is uninhibited, the response is one of toe flexion at the metatarso-phalangeal joints and may spread to the other foot. The bulbo-cavernosus reflex consists of contraction of the anal sphincter in response to squeezing of the glans penis. Both this manoeuvre and stroking of the perianal skin may evoke contraction of other muscles of sacral innervation, e.g. lateral hamstrings and foot intrinsics. The extent of the S2–4 dermatomes in the saddle area has been illustrated in Fig. 11.1.

Information on bladder function can be obtained more directly by simple observation and suprapubic pressure. The normal infant is not incontinent but passes urine at intervals in a proud, parabolic stream. Continuous dribbling on crying or suprapubic pressure is strongly suggestive of some kind of neurogenic bladder disorder.

Bowel. Although detailed correlative studies have not been carried out, S2–4 activity in the lower limbs appears to bear a similar relationship to bowel function as it does to bladder function. Again, constant leakage of

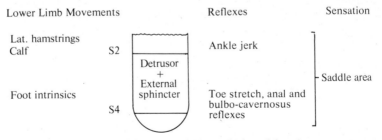

FIG. 11.2. Clinical signs of S2–4 spinal cord function.

meconium from a patulous anal sphincter is a warning of later problems in faecal continence.

SPECIAL INVESTIGATION

In neonatal assessment there is no need for elaborate investigation and no place for procedures such as ventriculography which may impair the infant's fitness for early surgery. The following procedures have, however, proved valuable.

(a) Bacteriological culture of swabs from the umbilicus and myelomeningocele.

(b) Radiological examination of skull, spine and hips. By taping sterile wire markers, e.g. pipe cleaners, around the lesion, its vertebral extent can be determined with greater accuracy (Fig. 11.3). Detection of unsuspected vertebral anomalies such as hemivertebrae and diastematomyelia may influence the decision to operate or the surgical technique which is employed. These initial films also provide a valuable base line for later reassessment, e.g. of hip or spinal deformity.

(c) Clinical photographs of the back lesion and lower limbs can be recommended for the same reason.

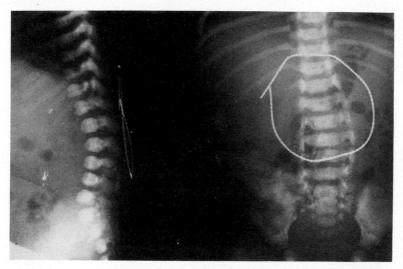

FIG. 11.3. X-ray spine showing myelomeningocele outlined by wire marker (T11–L4); on lateral film, note loss of anterior notching of vertebral bodies, opposite myelomeningocele.

Electrophysiological techniques in the first 24 hours of life are of mainly research interest. Direct faradic stimulation of the lesion is occasionally helpful in establishing whether a bare area in the sac includes neural tissue: contraction of lower limb muscles following stimulation suggests that the lesion is an open rather than a closed myelomeningocele and that the tissue in question must be treated with the greatest respect at operation. Although it has been advocated in neonatal assessment by Stoyle (1966), faradic stimulation is inferior to careful clinical examination in distinguishing 'voluntary' from purely reflex activity. In this regard, electromyography is of greater value, but has its main application at a later stage in guiding orthopaedic management and in the investigation of neurological deterioration.

Chapter 12

Closure of the Back

The first step in surgical management of myelomeningocele is closure of the back lesion. The most difficult step, however, is the decision to undertake operation.

Decision to Operate

If a policy of routine operation is followed, the assessment which has been described will be of value in predicting the child's later problems and in planning their solution. If, on the other hand, a selective approach is favoured, it will provide the facts on which the decision to operate can be based. Even if selection is accepted, opinion is likely to vary on what degree of handicap in survivors is unacceptable, i.e. on the stringency of selection criteria. If criteria are not strict and exclude only 20 per cent from active treatment, the proportion of severely handicapped survivors is likely to be high. If, on the other hand, we were to adopt very stringent criteria, for example, to exclude all infants with bladder involvement, the final results would be vitiated by survival of many untreated patients. Selection criteria must, therefore, be chosen which will strike a balance between the two extremes. The following are generally agreed to be major adverse features which are readily recognizable at birth and are present singly or in combination in 50–60 per cent of unselected infants with myelomeningocele.

1. Severe paralysis: voluntary motor level L3 or above.
2. Spinal deformity: severe kyphosis or scoliosis.
3. Gross hydrocephalus: OFC >2 cm above 90th percentile.
4. Major associated defects, e.g. cyanotic congenital heart disease, intestinal atresia, severe asphyxia or extreme prematurity.

Other criteria have been advocated from time to time but cannot be recommended without reservations. There is no doubt, as noted by Lorber (1972) that thoracolumbar and thoracolumbosacral lesions carry a particularly bad prognosis. Since, however, occasional infants with high lesions escape serious neurological involvement it is probably safer to base a decision on the observable effects of the lesion on the

81

lower limbs than on its level alone. There is very limited evidence to support the use of sensory level (Hunt *et al.*, 1973) and the presence of lacunar skull deformity (Stein *et al.*, 1974) as important selection criteria.

Selection criteria including those listed above should not be regarded as rigid and inviolable. A combination of adverse factors each just short of those defined may be no less predictive of severe disability than a single major criterion. Still stricter selection criteria may be appropriate in a developing country with more limited medical, educational and other resources for the handicapped. While the decision to operate should be determined mainly by the results of assessment of the child, major adverse social factors such as illegitimacy can be equally relevant to the outcome and cannot be ignored.

Consideration of social factors in selecting for operation is as controversial as is the extent to which the feelings and wishes of parents should influence the decision. De Lange (1974) considers that the interests of the patient alone should be taken into account and that the doctor's role should be as the patient's advocate. Since, however, it is the parents who will have to face the problems of caring for the child whose survival has been extended by surgery, it can equally well be argued that the decision should not be a purely medical one. Ellis (1974), for example, argues for direct parental involvement in decision making and sees the doctor as the parents' adviser.

In Edinburgh, a procedure has evolved which is a compromise between purely medical and exclusively parental decision. Following assessment and discussion among medical and surgical members of the team, a provisional decision is reached about the desirability of operation on the basis of the criteria which have been outlined. The paediatrician then discusses the situation with the child's father or, if possible, both parents. If assessment has revealed major adverse criteria, their practical significance is explained and the point made that, even with operation, the child's prospects of long-term survival would be poor. The parents are told that the baby can be kept in hospital and spared from suffering; the unlikely possibility of prolonged survival without operation is, however, mentioned. In the absence of major adverse criteria, on the other hand, the possibility of operation is explained; its limitations are emphasized and the child's future problems outlined as clearly as possible. They are reassured that help will be available at every stage and that each step in management will be fully explained. They are informed that although operation cannot make their child completely normal, without it he could still survive with increased disability.

Parents are not asked directly to make the final decision. As the choice concerns the lesser of two evils, neither option can be completely right. If they were to decide against operation, they might forever be haunted by the rejection of their own child; if they were to opt for surgical treatment they might be no less regretful when confronted by the reality of the child's disability. It is felt, therefore, that the burden of decision should rest on the doctors rather than the parents. The decision must, however, take account of parental feelings and attitudes to the handicapped which may emerge during the discussion, particularly in borderline cases. Parents are usually only too ready to accept 'whatever the doctor thinks best': the onus is, therefore, on the medical team to ensure that consent for operation is not a formality but based on a clear understanding of what is likely to be involved.

Ideally, the family doctor who is most familiar with the domestic situation and the parents' emotional resources should share in the process of decision. Although there may be practical difficulties, every effort should be made to involve him at least in the more difficult borderline cases.

At this point, management of the child selected for active treatment diverges from that of the child selected for purely symptomatic care. Management of the later will be outlined before the first steps in active treatment are considered.

The 'Untreated' Child

To be told that nothing can be done to help her malformed baby is distressing for any mother; to be asked to care for him at home as his condition steadily deteriorates and his back wound suppurates is the unkindest cut of all. With few exceptions, therefore, infants who are not given active treatment should be nursed in the paediatric unit. Further investigation such as ventriculography is unnecessary and the emphasis should be placed on minimizing distress. The following are offered as guidelines to practical management:

(a) normal nursing in a cot including regular sterile dressing of the myelomeningocele;

(b) feeding on demand with a full-strength formula but avoidance of nasogastric or parenteral nutrition;

(c) effective analgesia, e.g. with diamorphine, in the event of irritability associated with infection, but no antibiotic therapy;

(d) ventricular puncture to relieve distress related to raised intracranial pressure.

It is easier for the doctor to be objective about selective treatment than it is for the nurse who has to feed and handle the untreated infant, an infant who may look no different from the one receiving intensive treatment and who may look her in the eye and even smile as she nurses him. It is essential, therefore, that nurses given this difficult task should fully understand the reasons for withholding active treatment and be supported by an experienced ward sister and medical staff. With adequate explanation, however, even in units which have previously practised routine operation, nurses have been able to accept the desirability of selective treatment (Collis, 1972).

The extent to which parents visit and maintain contact with untreated infants varies considerably and is probably best left to them to decide. During the phase of mourning which may precede the child's death and which may be prolonged, they require continuing support from the social worker and family doctor. As they may hesitate to ask, they must be given reliable genetic counselling in the paediatric unit and the family doctor appraised of what they have been told (see Chapter 23).

With the conservative approach which has been outlined the overwhelming majority of these infants will die within the first 3 months of life (Hide et al., 1972; Stark and Drummond, 1973; Lorber, 1973). Unless, however, measures are employed which amount to frank euthanasia, the occasional infant will survive to 6 months or more. If the myelomeningocele becomes epithelialized and long-term survival is a real possibility, there should be no hesitation in inserting a shunt to control progressive hydrocephalus and subsequently managing the child as one of the selected group. As the untreated child has usually little to lose in terms of neurological function in the lower limbs and bladder, survival with increased disability can in this way be avoided. In such cases, parental acceptance of the child may, however, have been jeopardized. Nevertheless, in our experience, institutional care has very rarely been required.

Back Closure

Timing and Technique

There is no evidence that emergency back closure leads to improvement in lower limb function or even prevents the acute neurological deterioration which may occur within hours of birth (Stark and Baker, 1967; Brocklehurst et al., 1966; Smyth et al., 1974). Operation after the age of 48 hours is, however, followed by greater mortality and poorer quality of survival (Heimburger, 1972). If a decision has been taken to operate, it is, therefore, recommended that the back should be closed within 24–36 hours of birth. In the case of a closed myelomeningocele there is less urgency but no advantage in delaying operation.

Lorber and Bruce (1963) have shown that prophylactic chemotherapy is of no value but culture of a swab from the neural plate can provide a useful guide to chemotherapy in the event of post-operative infection.

The myelomeningocele can be repaired under local anaesthesia and sedation (for which purpose Heimburger, 1972, recommends whisky!). Most paediatric surgeons prefer general anaesthesia which is well tolerated by the newborn infant. The techniques of back closure have been well described and illustrated by Smith (1965) and Zachary and Sharrard (1967). The main steps in operation are separation of the neural plate from surrounding skin and membrane, exploration of the spinal canal for lesions which may tether or compress the cord, replacement of neural tissue in the spinal canal and secure closure of dura and skin.

If a selective policy is pursued, serious technical problems are unusual. If, however, the more extensive thoracolumbar lesions are tackled, major obstacles may have to be overcome. Direct closure of a very wide lesion may be impossible without excessive tension: relaxing incisions in the flanks or rotation of skin flaps may be necessary. Prominent everted laminae which are likely to cause pressure necrosis of overlying skin may have to be fractured and inverted to allow skin closure (Mustardé, 1966). In infants with severe kyphosis, closure may be possible only after the heroic procedure of vertebral osteotomy (Sharrard, 1968).

Post-operative Care

Following operation the infant should be nursed in an incubator prone or on his side to avoid pressure on the wound. If there is a danger of skin necrosis after closure of a large lesion, he can be held in ventral suspension from the roof of his incubator in a sling designed to relieve tension on the suture line (Zachary and Sharrard, 1967). The wound can be left exposed, but if it involves the sacral region it is better protected from faecal contamination by a dressing covered with a waterproof adhesive plaster such as 'Sleek'. Post-operative urinary retention may require relief by catheterization.

Early Complications

Post-operative problems are most likely to be encountered in infants whose lesions have been ruptured before operation, difficult to close or repaired after 36 hours.

Wound breakdown may occur from excessive tension in skin sutures or necrosis at the apex of rotation flaps. Healing will generally take place by granulation but split skin grafting may be necessary if the defect is large. If a leak of cerebrospinal fluid is the cause of wound breakdown, it will usually be necessary to reclose the dura and reduce ventricular pressure (see Chapter 13).

Wound infection is particularly likely to follow wound breakdown and is usually due to coliform organisms or less commonly *Staphylococcus pyogenes*. In view of the serious danger of spread to CSF pathways, prompt and effective systemic chemotherapy is essential. Pending culture and sensitivity reports, the treatment of choice is a combination of gentamicin 5 mg/Kg/day or kanamycin 15 mg/Kg/day with cloxacillin 50 mg/Kg/day intramuscularly. The child must be carefully observed for signs of meningitis such as head retraction and CSF cultured if there is any suspicion.

Meningitis

Even after early back closure, between 10 and 25 per cent of patients develop meningitis (Shurtleff, 1973). The most vulnerable are infants who have had a ruptured myelomeningocele or breakdown and infection of the back wound. Since infection reaches the CSF pathways through the myelomeningocele or back wound, *E. coli* and other Gram-negative organisms are usually responsible. *Staphylococcus pyogenes* and other Gram-positive bacteria are involved in about one-third. If the hydrocephalus is of communicating type, there will be an associated ventriculitis. In internal hydrocephalus, however, infection may not reach the lateral ventricles and be confined to the spinal meninges. In the former, ventricular CSF is of diagnostic value while in the latter it may be misleading.

The early clinical features are commonly non-specific, e.g. pyrexia and poor feeding. The infant may be pale or jaundiced, irritability is common and there may be signs of raised intracranial pressure, such as a tense fontanelle. Later developments are head retraction, convulsions and lesions of the lower cranial nerves. The child is particularly ill in Gram-negative infections in which collapse and septicaemia may occur.

Differential diagnosis is mainly from uncomplicated progressive hydrocephalus in which pyrexia and systemic illness are less frequent. Any suspicion of meningitis, however, is an indication for examination of CSF, which can most conveniently be obtained by puncture of the right lateral ventricle through the angle of the fontanelle. The characteristic features are an increase in cell count with polymorphs predominating, increased protein level and reduced or absent glucose. Gram-stained film and culture will identify the causative organism and sensitivity. If, despite evidence of meningitis, ventricular CSF is normal, there should be no hesitation in proceeding to careful cisternal or lumbar puncture to exclude isolated spinal meningitis.

In treating such a damaging infection, there is no place for half measures. A bactericidal level of the appropriate antibiotic must be achieved and maintained in CSF. As the blood-brain barrier in infancy is relatively impermeable to the newer antibiotics, chemotherapy must be given not only systemically but directly into the CSF pathways (Stark, 1967). For most Gram-negative infections, the drug of choice is gentamicin 5 mg/Kg/24 hours intramuscularly and 3–6 mg/24 hours by intraventricular injection depending on the degree of hydrocephalus.

Cisternal or intrathecal injection is, however, essential in spinal meningitis with clear ventricular fluid. Until bacteriological diagnosis has been established, cloxacillin 100 mg/Kg/24 hours intramuscularly and 10–20 mg/24 hours intraventricularly should also be given to cover the possibility of staphylococcal infection. In administration of intraventricular and intrathecal therapy, the drug should be drawn up in a 10 ml syringe and well diluted with CSF to facilitate its dispersal. Chemotherapy should be continued for at least 7–10 days and until three successive negative CSF cultures have been obtained. Eradication of infection should be confirmed a week after withdrawal of chemotherapy and prior to definitive shunt operation. CSF protein level may remain elevated for several weeks following clinical and bacteriological recovery.

If infection is slow to clear or recurrent, chemotherapy may have to be prolonged for several weeks. During this time, and even longer if CSF protein level is very high, insertion of a CSF shunt is precluded but control of hydrocephalus may be required. Appropriate measures are described in Chapter 13.

In addition to the above measures, the infant may require supportive therapy for peripheral circulatory failure or convulsions. Since ventriculitis is likely to be accompanied by cerebral oedema and foramen magnum coning, there is justification for adding dexamethasone 1–2 mg 6-hourly to the treatment regimen for the first few days (Stark, 1972b).

Shurtleff (1973) reported that even with active treatment only 57 per cent survived meningitis and only 50 per cent of survivors did well thereafter. Similarly, at follow-up, meningitis and valve complications were found to account for much of the worst disability in a series of children who had been selected for early operation (Stark and Drummond, 1973). If, therefore, a child whose disability is already moderate or severe fails to respond promptly to treatment of meningitis, the advisability of persisting with therapy is open to question.

Chapter 13

Control of Hydrocephalus

Assessment

Diagnosis of hydrocephalus presents few problems. More difficult, however, and more important is identification of the infant with *progressive* hydrocephalus which will require surgical treatment. Both clinical and neuro-radiological assessment are required for this purpose.

CLINICAL ASSESSMENT

The maximum occipitofrontal circumference should be measured daily during the first admission and recorded weekly on a percentile chart. At the same time, the child should be watched for signs of raised intracranial pressure described in Chapter 7.

Air ventriculography is the procedure of choice for assessment of ventricular enlargement and identification of the site of obstruction. It is usually carried out in the second or third week of life when the back wound has healed, but is unnecessary in the small minority of infants who show no clinical signs of hydrocephalus. The procedure, described in detail by Milhorat (1972), requires no anaesthesia but the strictest aseptic technique is essential. Using a 20-gauge spinal needle, the right lateral ventricle is tapped through the anterior fontanelle and, when the infant has settled, ventricular pressure measured in the supine position. Twenty to fifty ml CSF is then replaced with air and films taken in standard positions which allow it to reach all accessible parts of the ventricular system. On the erect lateral film, the cerebral mantle is measured as the distance between the roof of the lateral ventricle and the inner surface of the skull or anterior fontanelle at the vertex, a distance normally exceeding 35 mm in the newborn. Typical air ventriculograms are illustrated in Fig. 13.1.

CSF examination should be carried out routinely to exclude infection and provide base-line values for cell count, glucose and protein levels. Two other tests are of value in detection of neuronal breakdown products which are suggestive of progressive hydrocephalus. These are examinations of centrifuged deposit for fat-laden macrophages (Chester *et al.,* 1971) and estimation of creatine phosphokinase (Drummond and Belton, 1972).

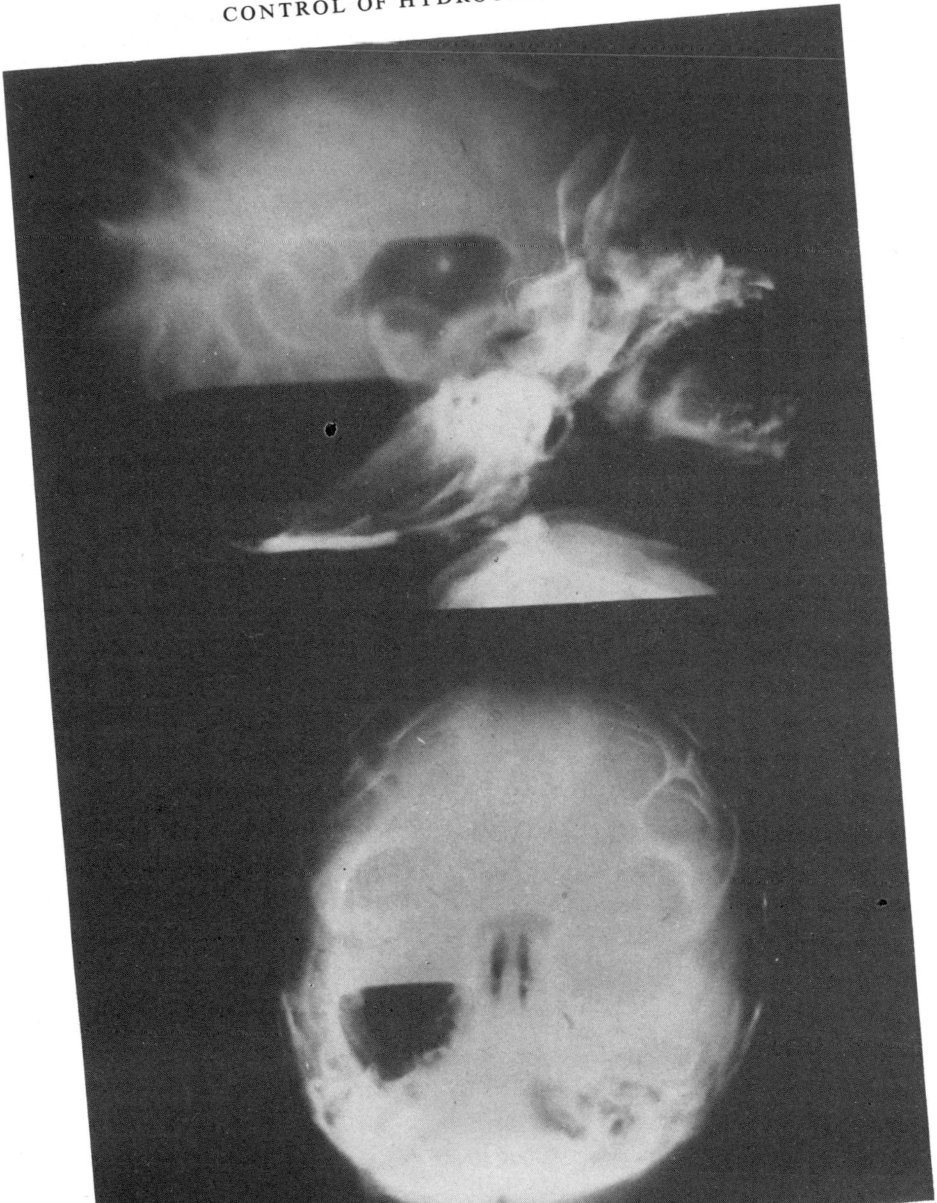

FIG. 13.1. Air ventriculograms. (a) Internal hydrocephalus due to aqueduct obstruction.

Other techniques. Positive contrast and *isotope ventriculography* are useful research techniques but offer no significant advantages in clinical practice. *Lumbar air encephalography* presents problems in infants with myelomeningocele and will, in any case, fail to delineate the ventricles in

aberrant distal catheter. Following emergency measures such as aspiration of the chest or pericardium, the distal catheter must be revised.

Infection. Infection is second to obstruction in incidence but presents greater problems in management. Two distinct syndromes will be considered: ventriculitis which is associated equally with ventriculoperitoneal and ventriculo-atrial shunts and septicaemia which results from colonization of the latter.

Ventriculitis, which may or may not be associated with meningitis, occurs in 10–12 per cent of patients with CSF shunts and is most likely to develop in the first 6 months of life. Infection is most commonly due to *Staphylococcus albus,* less often to *Staph. pyogenes* or Gram-negative organisms, introduced by ventricular puncture or at the time of shunt insertion. The *symptomatology* may simply be that of raised intracranial pressure due to ensuing obstruction of the ventricular catheter. Commonly, however, there is also fever, irritability, vomiting and head retraction. *Diagnosis* depends on examination and culture of ventricular CSF.

Since the implications of the label 'ventriculitis' are considerable it should not be attached to an infant uncritically. Isolation of *Staph. albus* from otherwise normal CSF can be due to contamination of the sample; in such circumstances, a second specimen should be obtained before committing the child to all that treatment involves. The main principles of *management* are removal of the shunt and sterilization of CSF followed by insertion of a new ventriculoperitoneal shunt (Stark, 1967). Combined systemic and intraventricular chemotherapy is necessary as recommended for neonatal meningitis (Chapter 11) with cloxacillin the drug of choice for infection with *Staph. albus.* After approximately 48 hours, the contaminated shunt is removed and its three components cultured. Insertion of a ventriculostomy reservoir at this stage facilitates intraventricular therapy and control of ventricular pressure. Chemotherapy is continued for 7–10 days and discontinued when three successive cultures have been negative. If, after a further 7–10 days, CSF remains sterile, the reservoir is removed and a new shunt inserted on the opposite side under antibiotic cover. If CSF protein content remains over 200 mg per cent, further delay is advised. Treatment along these lines is tedious and protracted but experience has taught the dangers of short cuts to eradication of ventriculitis.

Septicaemia is reported in 10–20 per cent of patients with ventriculo-atrial shunts (Luthardt, 1970; Morrice and Young, 1974). The underlying colonization of the shunt is usually with a particular *Staph. albus* (SIIA) which is well adapted to survival in Silastic® tubing by virtue of its ability to produce a protective film of mucus (Holt, 1969; Bayston and Penny, 1972). Organisms may gain access at the time of valve insertion or during transient bacteraemia at a later date (Holt, 1970; Bayston and

Lari, 1974). Antibiotic prophylaxis has, however, proved ineffective (Bayston, 1975).

The early *symptoms* which may be delayed for more than a year after operation are non-specific, e.g. malaise, pallor and low-grade pyrexia. The shunt continues to function but pumping it may be followed by a 'spike' of temperature. Anaemia gradually increases and the spleen becomes enlarged. *Diagnosis* depends on the finding of repeatedly positive blood cultures associated with sterile ventricular CSF (if ventricular fluid is infected, the condition is classified and treated as ventriculitis). *Treatment* is based on systemic and intraventricular chemotherapy (usually with cloxacillin) and removal of the colonized shunt after 48 hours. At the same operation, as ventricular fluid is sterile, a new *ventriculoperitoneal* shunt can be inserted incorporating a ventriculostomy reservoir through which cloxacillin can be injected for the following 7 days (Perrin and McLaurin, 1967). Although McLaurin and Dodson (1971) have shown that in a proportion of cases infection can be eradicated by massive intraventricular chemotherapy without shunt replacement, their revised policy has not yet found wide acceptance.

Decompression effects. Subdural haematoma is a rare complication of rapid decompression of ventricles under high pressure (Foltz and Shurtleff, 1963). In about 1 per cent of patients, long-term ventricular decompression results in craniostenosis from premature fusion of the sutures (Roberts and Rickham, 1970).

Remote complications. The occurrence of complications remote from the shunt itself is a particular hazard of the ventriculo-atrial operation and a cogent argument in favour of ventriculoperitoneal shunting. *Massive pulmonary embolism* with a high mortality rate from right ventricular failure can result from dislodgement of thrombus from the atrial catheter or a damaged tricuspid valve (Sperling *et al.*, 1964).

Chronic pulmonary hypertension results from more gradual silting up of the pulmonary vascular bed with small emboli. This phenomenon has been demonstrated in asymptomatic patients by lung scan (Brisman *et al.*, 1970) and in no fewer than 93 per cent at autopsy (Emery and Hilton, 1961). Its long-term clinical significance is still uncertain.

Shunt nephritis, reviewed by Meadow (1973), is a complication of *Staph. albus* colonization and septicaemia. It appears to result from deposition of immune complex in the glomeruli rather than bacterial embolization. A nephrotic syndrome is the usual clinical picture but hypertension and haematuria may also occur. When associated with the systemic effects of septicaemia, it may be mistaken for acute pyelonephritis. With the treatment outlined above resolution of the renal lesion can be expected in a few months.

Results of Treatment

The success of treatment can be measured by the control (or arrest) of hydrocephalus and the neurological integrity found in survivors.

Control of hydrocephalus, i.e. prevention of abnormal increase in head circumference, ventricular size and pressure, can be achieved in the vast majority of patients apart from temporary setbacks during episodes of CNS infection. The cost of control is a high incidence of life-threatening complications and perpetuation of shunt-dependency.

In an unknown proportion of patients, however, true *arrest of hydrocephalus* probably occurs so that even after blockage or removal of the shunt it ceases to progress. Mechanisms of arrest could include atrophy of the choroid plexus, increased transependymal escape of CSF or spontaneous drainage of the lateral ventricle into the subarachnoid space. As it is difficult to be certain that a shunt is totally without function, it is safer not to remove it. At the same time, however, if the child remains well there is no indication for revision of a blocked shunt.

Assessment of the *neurological results* of treatment is impeded by the multiplicity of variables involved: initial severity of hydrocephalus, selection for treatment, delay before shunting, incidence of complications, etc. Without selection, however, approximately 70 per cent of survivors should be in the normal range of intelligence (Lorber, 1971a). By avoiding operation in those with gross hydrocephalus at birth, even better results can be achieved in survivors (Stark and Drummond, 1973). Even with sparing of intelligence, however, subtle yet significant neurological deficits are very common. These long-term problems have been outlined in Chapter 8.

Chapter 14

Discharge Home

The chief objectives of the first admission are closure of the myelo-meningocele, control of hydrocephalus and *early discharge to the care of parents who are fully prepared and confident of continuing support.*

Early Discharge

In the absence of complications, it is possible to allow the infant home 2–3 weeks after birth. Problems such as wound breakdown or ventriculitis, however, may stretch the first admission into months. In the interests of early discharge we no longer carry out full assessment of the urinary tract during the first admission but readmit the child for a few days at 2–3 months when, in any case, the investigations are easier.

Preparation of Parents

Careful preparation of parents for the child's management at home is no less important than skilful surgical treatment of the infant. The main needs of parents at this stage will now be summarized briefly.

(a) *Reassurance.* After the negative feelings of loss, guilt and inadequacy which are likely to have followed their child's birth, parents are in particular need of positive reassurance. They require reassurance that nothing they have done or failed to do could have caused the infant's malformation; reassurance that although the problems are multiple, each will be explained with frankness and dealt with in turn as the need arises. Above all they need reassurance that their child's basic needs are the same as those of any other baby and that with the help which will be forthcoming, they will be able to cope.

(b) *Contact with the child.* The importance of the first few days of life in forging a normal attachment between mother and child has been emphasized by recent studies of Klaus *et al.* (1972). By simply allowing an extra 16 hours of contact with the child in the first 3 days of life, an appreciable effect on mothering could be demonstrated. In stark contrast is the report by Freeston (1971) that one-third of mothers of infants with spina bifida had never picked them up before taking them home from hospital. If acceptance of the child is to be fostered, mothers must be encouraged, even in the first week, to visit, feed and handle their infants in hospital.

(c) *Practical guidance.* During the first admission, parents should be given experience not only of routine everyday care but of any more specialized tasks which may be necessary, e.g. testing of a CSF shunt, bladder expression if recommended (but see Chapter 15), simple exercises, etc. If the mother can 'live in' for a few days she can acquire confidence in all aspects of her child's management while advice and assistance are readily available.

(d) *Genetic counselling.* Since they may hesitate to ask for it, all parents who have had an infant with myelomeningocele should be offered genetic counselling. The optimal timing is probably within a month of the child's birth although the information given may have to be repeated or clarified later. In the immediate postnatal period, however, when parents are already suffering from a barrage of unwelcome information, genetic counselling is likely only to compound their confusion with feelings of guilt. Although there are now genetic advice centres in the larger areas of population, counselling is probably more appropriately provided by the paediatrician who has already developed a close rapport with parents. He will, moreover, be conversant with the local treatment policy which would affect the outcome for a second affected child. Details of recurrence risks and methods of antenatal diagnosis are discussed in Chapter 23. Whether genetic advice is given by a paediatrician or geneticist it is essential that the family doctor, social worker and health visitor should know exactly what parents have been told so that any confusion can be avoided.

(e) *Emotional support.* The feelings and behaviour of parents of a severely handicapped child have been set out with unsurpassed clarity by MacKeith (1973). Parents may find it difficult to express feelings, especially of anger, guilt and rejection to a doctor directly concerned with treatment of their child. A medical social worker, in possession of the facts of the child's case, is in a strategic position to listen to their worries and fears, to relay unanswered questions to the paediatrician and provide continuing emotional support. For some parents support of this kind can be provided also by the family doctor or minister who have the advantage of a prior relationship with the family. Their constructive involvement, however, depends on a continuing supply of information on the child's condition and prospects.

Liaison with Community Services

If they are to contribute substantially to management so that complete dependence on the specialist hospital can be avoided, the family doctor, community social worker, health visitor and physiotherapist must be informed in advance of the child's discharge home. A brief telephone contact is worth more than a three-page summary which arrives 3 weeks later. Ideally, however, they should be invited to visit the paediatric unit before the child's discharge to meet their hospital counterparts, discuss the next steps in management and become identified by parents as an extension of the hospital team. In this way it has been found that the parents' trust in the health visitor and consequently her contribution to the child's care can be greatly enhanced.

Copies of the discharge summary which should outline not only what has been done to the child but what has been said to parents, should be sent to all members of the medical/surgical team and to those in the community whose assistance is to be recruited. This early communication with the Department of Community Medicine should result in the child's inclusion in the handicap register.

Follow-up

Organization of hospital follow-up has been described in Chapter 10. The first follow-up visit should be within 2–3 weeks of discharge and parents reassured that, in the meantime, they should not hesitate to telephone the paediatrician, ward sister or medical social worker should problems arise.

Prevention and Treatment of Urinary Tract Infection

PREVENTION

Prevention of infection depends, above all, on reduction of residual urine by relief of bladder outlet obstruction, prevention of severe constipation and regular manual expression if the detrusor is feeble. A large fluid intake and urine output may prevent organisms in the bladder reaching the 'climax' population associated with infection – a fact requiring emphasis to parents who are inclined to restrict the fluid intake of an incontinent child. There is no evidence that prophylactic chemotherapy is of any value (Lorber *et al.,* 1967). Long-term administration of sulphonamides and ampicillin which have a profound effect on intestinal flora may be harmful by encouraging colonization with highly resistant organisms. Winberg (1973) advocates the application of an antiseptic cream to the urethral meatus to prevent ascent of faecal organisms but offers no evidence of its efficiency.

DIAGNOSIS

In the clinical picture of urinary infection in these patients, urinary symptoms are seldom conspicuous although parents may have noted an increase in dribbling incontinence, unusually offensive urine or excoriation of the perineum. Symptomatology is usually non-specific. There may be a fulminating illness with endotoxin shock from Gram-negative septicaemia; more often, there is simply malaise, fever and vomiting which may suggest a blocked shunt or ventriculitis. Not infrequently, urinary infection is completely asymptomatic.

Diagnosis depends on urine culture not only in the presence of suggestive symptoms but as a routine every 3 months if the child has a neurogenic bladder. It is even more difficult to lay down strict diagnostic criteria for urinary infection than in children without neurogenic bladders. It is customary to regard a colony count of 10^6 per ml in a freshly cultured CCU as evidence of infection, which is strengthened if there are clumps of pus cells on microscopy. In doubtful cases, e.g. counts of 10^5 per ml and mixed growths, bladder stab can provide decisive information: a bacterial count of even 10^3 per ml in such a specimen is strongly suggestive of infection.

If urine culture is indicated more often than the child attends the spina bifida clinic, arrangements can usually be made for reliable specimens to be collected in the health centre or surgery for culture in the district hospital. Parents living in remote areas can be taught to use dipslides such as Uricult ®, which can then be sent by post to hospital for colony counting and subculture (Arneil *et al.,* 1973). A separate sheet in the child's case folder has proved useful in follow-up for tabulation of bacterial species, colony count, sensitivity, recommended treatment and side-effects.

TREATMENT

During episodes of infection a high fluid intake is more important than ever. In the past, prolonged courses of antibiotics have been recommended in the belief that relapse would occur from emergence of organisms which had survived a shorter period of chemotherapy. It is now generally accepted that relapse of this kind is much rarer than reinfection with a different organism (Bergström et al., 1967). Although long-term chemotherapy may prevent reinfection in anatomically normal children (Normand and Smellie, 1965), there is, as noted above, no evidence that it does so in patients with neurogenic bladder disorders. There would, therefore, appear to be no advantage in continuing chemotherapy for more than 10–14 days. Following treatment, cultures should be repeated monthly and reinfection treated for a similar period.

TABLE 15.1. Chemotherapy of urinary tract infection.

Drug	Dosage mg/kg/24 hr	Frequency	Route
Ampicillin	50	6 hourly	oral, IM, IV
Carbenicillin	200	6 hourly	IM, IV
Cephalexin	50	6 hourly	oral
Cephaloridine	50	8 hourly	IM, IV
Colistin	2·5–5	8 hourly	IM, IV
Cotrimoxazole			
trimethoprin	2	12 hourly	oral
sulphamethoxazole	10		
Gentamicin	3–6	8 hourly	IM, IV
Kanamycin	15	12 hourly	IM
Nalidixic acid	50	6 hourly	oral
Nitrofurantoin	5	6 hourly	oral
Sulphadimidine	150	6 hourly	oral

The choice of chemotherapy depends on the infecting organism, most commonly *Esch. coli* or *Proteus*, and its sensitivity. The more commonly used drugs and their dosage are listed in Table 15.1, ampicillin, sulphadimidine and co-trimoxazole are the drugs of choice for sensitive organisms. More toxic drugs which require parenteral administration (e.g. gentamicin, colistin) and more expensive drugs (e.g. cephalexin) should be reserved for the attack on *Pseudomonas pyocyanea* and other resistant organisms. Low grade pseudomonas infection in the bladder or in an ileal conduit may be cleared by irrigation with a solution of colistin (500 000 units in 20 ml normal saline).

Reassessment of the Urinary Tract

Even if the child appears to have a safe bladder, careful follow-up studies are essential to detect the earliest signs of deterioration. At each clinic visit, i.e. at least 3-monthly in the first year, the bladder should be palpated and, if expression has been advised, the ease with which this can be carried out assessed. At the same time, a 'clean-catch' urine specimen is obtained for culture. Blood pressure should be recorded at least annually in the school age child.

Every 12–18 months, it is our practice to admit the child for 2–3 days for further assessment of the urinary tract. Unless there has been an appreciable change in the neurological picture, there is no need to repeat bladder pressure studies. Intravenous pyelography can also be omitted unless deterioration is suggested by the isotope renogram which is more sensitive and entails much less radiation. Micturating cysto-urethrography, urine cultures and biochemical studies are, however, routine and the admission provides an opportunity for assessment of bladder control.

If the bladder remains safe and upper urinary tract normal, conservative management is continued. Increasing outlet obstruction or developing hydronephrosis may, however, occasionally necessitate surgical intervention as described earlier.

Control of Incontinence

Although readily accepted in the first 2 or 3 years of life, urinary incontinence looms increasingly large as school age approaches. In the absence of an ideal solution, it is wise to begin with simple conservative measures for its control. If they succeed, urinary diversion may be avoided; if they fail, its necessity is likely to be more easily accepted by parents.

BLADDER TRAINING
The child whose bladder function is considered to be normal on initial assessment should be potty-trained in the normal way. Too much should, however, not be expected from 'training' of the child who simply does not have the neurological apparatus for normal bladder control. In the view of Eckstein (1968), if continence is not achieved by the age of 3 years it is unlikely to develop later. Although this may apply to complete continence, a useful measure of 'social continence' – the ability to be dry for more than 3 hours without appliances – may be obtained much later in childhood. The training régime which depends on enthusiasm and perseverance consists of regular bladder emptying at intervals of 1 hour or less, increasing with success to 3 or 4 hours. In the young child the mother carries out manual expression provided that it has been shown to be safe. As the child grows older, he is encouraged to strain and later assist with manual expression.

In the early stages of training, Nergårdh et al. (1974) who have an enviable record of success recommend a very high fluid intake and carefully selected drug therapy as an adjunct to expression and straining. They give carbachol injections to induce autonomous detrusor contractions in inert bladders and diazepam to reduce external sphincter spasm in patients with reflex bladders.

Initiation of these more intensive régimes of training unfortunately entails hospital admission for at least one month.

Portable urinals. No effective portable urinal has yet been devised for use in girls. Portable urinals are, however, worth a trial in boys who at the age of about 4 years are still dribbling between episodes of manual expression. Suitable appliances include the Heritage* urinal. Careful fitting, a service provided by some suppliers, is essential if both leakage and pressure ulceration of the penis are to be avoided. The mother is advised to cut a hole in the front of the child's underpants through which the appliance can pass. Manual expression is continued, the function of the urinal being to collect any intervening dribbles. The success of portable urinals varies greatly and doubtless owes much to the enthusiasm and conviction of the doctor. We have found it least satisfactory in boys confined to a wheelchair and, conversely, in those who have least physical handicap.

CATHETER DRAINAGE

The alternative to the often disappointing measures outlined has generally been urinary diversion which Smith (1972a) and other authorities still advocate as a more or less routine measure at the age of 2 years or less. When carried out simply to control incontinence, however, diversion implies sacrifice of competent ureteric orifices and an appreciable risk of deterioration of a previously normal upper urinary tract. In Smith's (1972b) series, 10 per cent of patients in whom IVP was normal before operation deteriorated after diversion and those with already dilated ureters deteriorated more often than they improved. Other authors have reported dilatation of 27·5 per cent and 42 per cent of previously normal ureters following diversion (Cook *et al.,* 1968; Susset *et al.,* 1966). For this reason, as well as the high incidence of practical problems associated with urinary diversion, there has recently been a reappraisal of indwelling catheter drainage in control of urinary incontinence (Duthie and Stark, 1974; Forrest, 1974).

In Edinburgh we have been favourably impressed by the new silicone-elastomer catheter (Silicath†) which needs to be changed only every 4–6 weeks. A size 14 French gauge Foley catheter is inserted at first, but

*Salt and Sons Ltd., 220 Corporation St., Birmingham.

†Travenol Laboratories Ltd., Thetford, Norfolk.

larger sizes are usually required to prevent leakage as the urethra becomes dilated. The catheter is drained into a 200 ml polyethylene bag* with a non-return valve or into a larger bag at night. When dryness has been achieved on continuous drainage, the catheter is spigotted and released at intervals increasing from 1–3 hours.

Experience to date suggests that good control of incontinence can be achieved in at least 60 per cent of cases and that infection and upper urinary tract damage are not serious dangers in the short term. Until the results of more prolonged follow-up studies are available, catheters can be recommended only on a trial basis and in children who can be closely monitored for infection and dilatation of the upper urinary tract.

URINARY DIVERSION

If, when the urinary tract is reassessed at 4–$4\frac{1}{2}$ years of age, incontinence remains a problem despite adequate trial of the above conservative measures, there is no socially acceptable alternative to diversion of the urinary stream. Since this is not only a major surgical procedure but a psychologically distressing one, both parents and child must be carefully prepared for it well in advance. They should not be led to expect absolute control of incontinence from the day of operation but to anticipate temporary difficulties in the early stages with the reassurance that practical help will be available. The parents will usually welcome the opportunity of seeing an older child with a satisfactory diversion and of discussing it with his parents. The doctor explaining the nature of the operation must remember that even well-informed adults have often only the vaguest notions of anatomy and physiology. Preparation of the child is even more difficult: pre-operative fitting of a diversion appliance is likely to be more meaningful than detailed anatomical description. The proposed diversion must be discussed also with the orthopaedic surgeon to ensure that positioning of the stoma will not prejudice future hip surgery or bracing.

If diversion is indicated mainly for control of incontinence, the ureters which are too short and narrow for ureterostomy must be inserted into an intestinal conduit which can be brought out through the abdominal wall to form a stoma to which a collecting bag can be fitted. Although loops of colon have been employed, most surgeons now prefer the ileal conduit operation described by Bricker (1950) and illustrated diagramatically in Fig. 15.4. Fashioning of the stoma so that it is neither flush with the skin nor too long, and strategic placing to avoid abdominal scars, creases and bony prominences are important points in surgical technique. Success depends also on meticulous attention to details of

*Bardic.

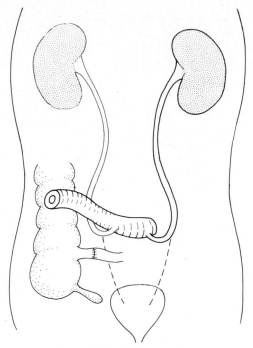

FIG. 15.4. Ileal loop diversion.

everyday management of the diversion about which parents require clear explanation and practical demonstration.

Many of the problems associated with the older rubber ileostomy bags have disappeared with introduction of disposable plastic appliances specifically designed for urinary diversion. Experience has proven the Carshalton* and Hollister† bags eminently satisfactory. The Hollister appliance is particularly simple to use as it is in one piece, i.e. a collecting bag with adhesive flange for attachment to the skin and lugs providing for the added security of a light body belt. To minimize excoriation of the skin by urine, the appliance should be selected with an opening no more than $\frac{1}{4}''$ greater in diameter than the stoma itself. For good adhesion, the skin must be clean and absolutely dry when the appliance is attached with the spout central in its aperture. In the active child, still greater security can be obtained by overlapping the edges of the flange with waterproof adhesive strapping. If sweating is marked, the skin under the bag should be powdered with talc. To ensure free drainage from the loop, the clothes should not be so tight as to compress the stoma.

*Eschmann Bros. and Walsh Ltd., 24 Church St., Shoreham-by-Sea, Sussex.

†Abbot Laboratories Ltd., Queenborough, Kent.

To prevent leakage, the bag should not be allowed to become more than half full. During the day it must, therefore, be emptied every 3–4 hours by release of a simple clamp. If the child attends a normal school, explanation of his problem to staff is necessary to ensure a measure of privacy in the lavatory and spare unnecessary embarrassment. The school nurse and hygiene aide are useful allies when available. At night, a plastic tube is used to connect the appliance to a larger bag or other suitable receptacle for the overnight urine. The watertight seal between appliance and skin will commonly survive bathing and swimming after which the wet belt must, of course, be changed. When, after a few days, the seal breaks down, the bag is gently removed and a new one fitted after careful cleaning of the stoma and surrounding skin.

In the early weeks after diversion operation, frustration and disappointment are common. If leakage occurs despite careful application of the appliance, its adhesion can be reinforced by coating the peristomal skin with Tinct. Benzoin. Co. or a proprietary aerosol adhesive.* Some parents are helped by the explanatory literature published by the appliance manufacturers. The practical handbook of Gibney (1970) is of value not only for parents but for their medical and nursing advisers. In the U.K., urinary diversion appliances are provided through the National Health Service and parents are asked to contact the children's hospital for order of a replacement set before their supply of bags runs out.

Like CSF shunts, urinary diversions are notoriously prone to complications. The incidence of potentially fatal *immediate complications* such as intestinal obstruction or infarction and wound dehiscence is still 10–20 per cent (Smith, 1972; Scott, 1973).

In approximately 25 per cent of patients an offensive urethral discharge occurs from chronic infection in the 'forgotten bladder'. If such *bladder empyema* relapses after four weekly irrigations with 1:1000 chlorhexidine, the most satisfactory answer is cystectomy (Eckstein and Mohindra, 1970).

Stomal complications are also common. Ulceration of the stoma which may lead to an intractable skin-level fistula is usually due to pressure from an appliance whose aperture is too small or eccentrically placed. Like a skin-level fistula, retraction, stenosis, overgrowth and herniation of the stoma are usually indications for surgical revision. Peristomal ammoniacal dermatitis is not uncommon and distinct from contact dermatitis which is clearly confined to the area of the flange. In such cases, a steroid cream should be applied until the skin has recovered and the adhesive changed. In patients with particularly sensitive skins, Karaya Gum washers are not only innocuous but provide a good seal.

*e.g. Hollister Medical Adhesive or Dow-Corning Medical Adhesive.

As already noted, there is a disquieting tendency for *dilatation of the upper urinary tract* to follow urinary diversion. The cause may be the ureteric reflux which usually occurs from ileal loops (Smith, 1972b) or elevation of pressure in the loop by pressure from clothing, orthopaedic appliances or sleeping in the prone position (Scott, 1973). Since uretero-ileal stenosis is an occasional cause, pyelographic evidence of hydroureter should prompt contrast x-ray study of the ileal loop.

Alternative diversion procedures have been used which have the advantage of retaining competent ureteric orifices. Cystostomy is now generally condemned (Ireland and Geist, 1970). Colocystostomy, in which a colonic loop attached to the bladder provides a more satisfactory stoma has also proved disappointing in practice. The latest operation of this type in which the bladder trigone is incorporated in an ileal conduit, ileo-trigonal diversion, has not yet been fully evaluated (Pond and Texter, 1970).

Other Approaches to Control of Incontinence

Justifiable dissatisfaction with conventional methods of treatment has stimulated a continuing search for alternatives. A few examples will be outlined to illustrate the diversity of approach to the difficult problem of urinary incontinence. None of these methods can, however, yet be recommended without reservation.

Detrusor stimulation. Habib (1963) and others have demonstrated satisfactory emptying of the bladder in paraplegic dogs by stimulation of a trigger area near the ureterovesical junction. Coordinated contraction of the human bladder is, however, less easily achieved and the implanted electrodes are prone to many complications (Halverstadt and Leadbetter, 1968; Caldwell, 1968).

Pelvic floor stimulation. The converse, continuous faradic stimulation of the pelvic floor (and external sphincter), has met with some success in adults with paraplegia or stress incontinence (Caldwell *et al.,* 1965; Hopkinson and Lightwood, 1967). Children with neurogenic bladders, however, who have a pelvic floor capable of responding to stimulation are commonly those whose upper urinary tract is already in danger from detrusor-sphincter dyssinergia. Implantation of pelvic floor stimulators has had very limited success in these patients (Caldwell *et al.,* 1969).

Endovesical electrotherapy. Katona (1958) has described a technique of stimulating the bladder per urethram which he claims capable of evoking more effective detrusor activity The rationale of the method which is very tedious for the child is obscure and there is nothing in recent reports to encourage more extensive trial (Eckstein, 1974).

Artificial sphincter. Scott *et al*. (1974), have recently developed a cuff which is implanted around the posterior urethra and can be inflated and deflated by the patient. It has been employed in children with spina bifida but adequate follow-up studies are still awaited.

Chapter 16

Control of Faecal Incontinence

The neurogenic bowel is perhaps the most underestimated problem associated with spina bifida. For the clinician, it is an uninviting affair which does not have the same medical significance as the neurogenic bladder. For parents, it is so embarrassing that they may hesitate to discuss it especially when the child is present. Consequently, they often receive little practical guidance and are left to find their own solutions to the problem (Woodburn, 1974).

Assessment

Assessment of the neurogenic bowel still lacks the sophistication of urinary tract assessment and cannot yet provide such a rational guide to management. It is, however, of some predictive value and merits further exploration. Clinical assessment must include a careful history to clarify whether the child has any rectal sensation and ability for voluntary evacuation. The history will usually indicate whether there is simply partial or complete lack of control or a problem of chronic constipation with overflow incontinence. Abdominal palpation and rectal examination are useful measures of constipation. Neurological attention should be directed to function, normal, absent or purely reflex, in S2–4 territory in the lower limbs as described on p. 78. The subcutaneous external sphincter is a pointer to activity in the functionally more important puborectalis sling. It can be assessed by simple observation and by elicitation of the anal and bulbocavernosus reflexes. These simple tests correlate well with measurements of tension and electrical activity in the external sphincter (Chantraine *et al.,* 1966). In doubtful cases, puborectalis function can be assessed directly by barium enemas as described by Tsuchida *et al.* (1972).

Techniques such as anorectal manometry have not yet found a place in routine assessment but are valuable in research and may yet provide a more physiological basis for management (White *et al., 1972).

Management

Principles
Whether the child has an inert or reflex type of bowel disorder, the following general principles of management apply:

1. prevent faecal retention and impaction which will not only lead to overflow incontinence but further reduce contractility of the recto-sigmoid;

2. if the colon is already impacted, ensure its complete evacuation as a first step;

3. aim for regular daily evacuation at a predictable time and before rectal distension evokes reflex defaecation or passively overcomes the internal sphincter.

Practice
In the first year of life, stools are soft and impaction less likely. Regular bladder expression will usually empty the rectum simultaneously.

From the second year, most patients will require some medication to ensure daily evacuation. Our methods of achieving this are based on the recommendations of Forsythe and Kinley (1970). In the first instance, Senokot syrup is given before the evening meal in a dosage of 5–10 ml. It is hoped that allied to the gastrocolic reflex it will stimulate defaecation about half an hour later when the child is 'potted' for 20 minutes. As the effect of Senokot is variable, timing and dosage must be adjusted to suit the individual child. For some, twice or thrice daily administration is required.

Continence is more easily achieved if the stools are formed but reasonably firm; those with the consistency of paste on the one hand or granite on the other are equally undesirable. By trial and error, mothers usually learn how the child's diet affects the stools and may be able to achieve the desired result without the use of medication. Antibiotics such as ampicillin given for urinary tract infection are likely to upset even the best-mannered bowel. Persistently hard stools can be softened with a preparation such as Dioctyl (Medo) syrup 5–10 ml t.i.d. well-diluted with water. Oily preparations such as liquid paraffin should be avoided as they tend to cause constant oozing especially in the child with inert rectum and pelvic floor.

If a day is missed, a suppository such as bisacodyl (Dulcolax®) 5 mg will usually secure an evacuation. The mother must be reminded not only to remove the silver paper from the suppository but to ensure that it is retained for long enough in the anorectal canal. If the external sphincter is lax, the child should be laid on his side with the buttocks held together for 20–30 minutes before he is placed on the pottie or w.c. for defaecation. Although entirely oral medication is preferable, some children require a suppository 2 or 3 times a week in addition.

If the bowel holds out against this siege for more than 2 days, more drastic measures must be deployed to prevent serious impaction. Manual evacuation is distasteful but effective. As an alternative, the mother or district nurse can administer a 'disposable' micro-enema such as Micralax (Smith, Kline and French).

If training is to be successful, the child must have no fears of his pottie, the lavatory or the process of defaecation. Such fears may be engendered if he is left alone, if he is placed on the pottie before he has developed good sitting balance or if his mother shows obvious impatience and anger when he fails to perform. The whole experience should be made as pleasant as possible; the child should be warm, comfortable and entertained. The mother should not expect success overnight but should be encouraged to show delight when the child obliges rather than frustration when he fails. Even in the preschool years, independence should be fostered. The child with rectal sensation should be rewarded when he recognizes the call to stool: the child with an inert bowel should be encouraged to strain with his abdominal muscles when sitting on the pottie. Later, he can, if necessary, be given a supply of disposable plastic gloves and taught to insert a suppository without assistance. Every effort should be made to avoid a long-term régime of manual evacuation or enemas which not only foster dependence but have potentially adverse psychological effects (Riveille, 1962).

Until 'accidents' are infrequent and soiling negligible, the child will usually have to wear disposable nappies or incontinence pads which are available on NHS prescription. Deodorants may increase the child's confidence at school, and to prevent soiling on important social occasions a vaginal tampon can be inserted in the anorectal canal.

Special Problems

Faecal impaction. If the child presents late or if, despite the measures outlined, increasing constipation supervenes, with constant leakage of liquid faeces from a loaded rectum, hospital admission is usually required. After the bowel has been completely emptied by daily enemas for 5–10 days, a programme of oral medication is introduced before discharge.

Rectal prolapse. This infrequent complication tends to occur in the inert bowel with lax anal sphincter and may be precipitated by repeated manual evacuations. If the condition does not resolve spontaneously satisfactory results can be obtained by amputation of the prolapsed bowel as described by Nash (1972).

Results

With enthusiasm and persistence, remarkably good results can be achieved by the simple measures which have been described. At least 50 per cent of patients should become completely clean and most of the remainder should have no more than faecal staining of the underclothing (Forsythe and Kinley, 1970; Scobie *et al.*, 1970; White *et al.*, 1972). Dissatisfaction with these results or with the effort required to achieve them has continued to stimulate a search for alternatives which will now be outlined.

Other Methods of Treatment

Colostomy has been employed but is now generally condemned in these patients as unnecessarily drastic and itself a cause of further problems.

Pelvic floor stimulation. In 1967, Hopkinson and Lightwood reported their experience of electrical stimulation of the pelvic floor through electrodes incorporated in a perspex anal plug. A measure of success was achieved in adults with rectal prolapse but no claims made for its efficacy in children with neurogenic bowel incontinence

Gracilis sling operation. Dickson and Nixon (1968) made another ingenious approach to the problem. A gracilis muscle with intact nerve supply was detached from its insertion and looped round the rectum to form an additional striated muscle sphincter. Continuous contraction of the muscle was obtained by stimulation of its motor point through an externally placed radio transmitter and subcutaneous receiver-stimulator. Results have, however, been very disappointing in spina bifida children who lack rectal sensation (Dickson, 1975).

Rectal electrotherapy. Katona and Eckstein (1974) have advocated electrical stimulation of the rectum analogous to their treatment for the neurogenic bladder. Stimulation is claimed to 'set up reflex contractions of the smooth muscle of the bowel wall' and to have an 'indirect regulating effect on the sphincter mechanism'. In a preliminary trial, complete recovery of bowel function was claimed in each of seven children with lumbosacral spina bifida. In view of the dubious physiological basis for this therapy, the results of more extensive trials can be awaited only with scepticism.

Chapter 17

Orthopaedics and Mobilization

When back closure and control of hydrocephalus have been achieved and any immediate threat from the neurogenic bladder averted, the child's locomotor disability demands increasing attention. This chapter is concerned with the general principles of orthopaedic management and mobilization rather than details of surgical treatment, for which the reader is referred to the admirable reviews of Menelaus (1971), Parsch and Schulitz (1972) and Sharrard (1973).

Assessment

The nature of the lower limb problem in myelomeningocele has been described in Chapter 5 and its assessment in Chapter 11. Neonatal neurological and orthopaedic assessment has several objectives.

Prediction of deformity. The type and severity of deformity which will later confront the orthopaedic surgeon can be predicted from the neurological level and pattern at birth. For example, the child with an L4 motor level is threatened with early dislocation of the hips and the patient with isolated function in S1–5 cord with spastic equinus and knee flexion deformities. Conversely, the orthopaedic surgeon who is involved in the neonatal period can anticipate the treatment which will be required and plan it in relation to other aspects of the child's care.

Prediction of walking ability. Other things being equal, the degree of ambulation which can be expected is related to the voluntary motor level as summarized in Table 17.1. The child's walking ability will, however, be influenced by other factors such as his intelligence and motivation, upper limb function, freedom from spinal deformity and the adequacy of treatment.

Base-line for re-assessment. In most infants with myelomeningocele, the neurological lesion has stabilized by the age of 3 months. *Functional*

TABLE 17.1.

Voluntary motor level	Probable walking ability
T12 or above	Entirely wheelchair
L1–3	Predominantly wheelchair
	Limited walking in long calipers
	+ walking aid
L4–S1	Walking in short calipers
	± walking aid
S2–5	Walking without appliances

deterioration in the lower limbs may still occur from the effects of growth, obesity and persisting muscle imbalance. True *neurological* deterioration such as ascent of the motor level or increasing lower limb spasticity is an indication for myelography and neurosurgical intervention if it reveals tethering of the spinal cord, diastematomyelia or progressive hydromyelia.

Early Management

In the first 6 months, management is generally conservative and its main objective to contain deforming forces until the time for definitive corrective surgery.

Physiotherapy. However skilful, the physiotherapist cannot be expected to correct deformity due to muscle imbalance. Regular passive movements which parents should be taught to carry out are, however, of value in maintaining joint range and can prevent postural deformities in totally paralysed limbs. Forceful stretching of anaesthetic, osteoporotic limbs must be avoided. Attempted abduction of the hips in the face of strong adductor muscles can lead to fracture of the femur, and other manoeuvres can lead to the kind of bony injuries found in the battered baby. The child should be given experience of different postures including prone lying, supported sitting and weight-bearing on the feet, if they are reasonably plantigrade.

Strapping and splinting. Continuous splinting should theoretically be able to present overstretching of weak muscles by powerful antagonists. With this in mind, Walker (1968) has recommended careful application of Elastoplast strapping to control paralytic equinovarus deformity, and McKibbin (1973) has devised a light abduction splint to delay flexion-adduction deformity of the hips. Attempts to correct paralytic deformity with rigid plaster casts are, however, to be condemned, and many orthopaedic surgeons prefer to avoid any kind of splinting in view of the vulnerability of anaesthetic skin.

Operative treatment is seldom required in the early months of life. There is, however, occasionally a case for tenotomy of an unopposed or spastic muscle which is expected to cause rapidly progressive deformity in the first year of life.

Correction of Deformity

Since deformity in myelomeningocele usually results from muscle imbalance, its correction depends on abolition of deforming forces and restitution of muscle balance at each joint. If paralytic deformity is present at more than one level, it is preferable to treat the proximal deformity first, e.g. to reduce dislocated hips before correction of the knees or feet. Ideally, all major deformities should be corrected and the feet made plantigrade before the age of 2 years. To illustrate the methods of rebalancing muscle power in the lower limbs, management of some of the commoner paralytic deformities will now be outlined.

Dislocation of the hip. The standard approach to this deformity is the posterior iliopsoas transfer developed by Sharrard (1964b) and carried out between 9 and 18 months. Following open adductor release and reduction of the dislocation, the iliopsoas muscle is detached from the insertion into the lesser trochanter, which ensures its activity as a flexor and adductor of the hip. It is re-routed through an artificial foramen in the iliac bone and inserted into the back of the greater trochanter so that, acting as an extensor and abductor, it will hold the femoral head in the acetabulum (Fig. 17.1). The child is immobilized in a hip spica for about 4 weeks following operation but can be allowed home before it is removed. With early iliopsoas transfer, acetabular development should remain normal. If, however, treatment has been delayed or dislocation recurs, a bony operation such as the Salter osteotomy may also be required to deepen the acetabulum.

In general, there is little to be gained by transferring a muscle with power of less than MRC 3. If dislocation is associated with weak hip flexor activity, e.g. in a child with L1–2 motor level, psoas tenotomy is usually sufficient to correct muscle imbalance. In such patients, who have coxa valga from lack of gluteal pull, improvement of the femoral neck-shaft angle by varus osteotomy will help to maintain reduction of the dislocation.

Genu recurvatum (Fig. 5.4). This deformity can be very striking in infants with unopposed quadriceps (L3–4 motor level). After gentle passive mobilization of the knee in the early months of life, the quadriceps is lengthened at the age of 12–18 months by the procedure of Curtis and Fisher (1969). This operation restores muscle balance by weakening

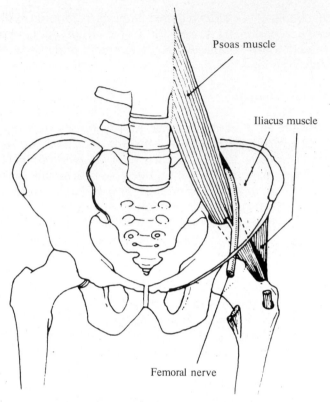

FIG. 17.1. Posterior ilio-psoas transplantation.

quadriceps and allowing sartorius and gracilis to function normally as flexors of the knee.

The recurvatum deformity which occurs from pressure on flail limbs which have been extended *in utero* does not require surgical treatment as there is no muscle imbalance. Caliper support will, however, be necessary after passive mobilization has been achieved.

Knee flexion deformity. Since the hamstrings have a lower segmental innervation than quadriceps, paralytic knee flexion deformity is not a feature of Type I neurological lesions but can occur in Type II lesions from hamstring spasticity. The power of the hamstrings as knee flexors can be reduced without loss of their hip extensor activity by transfer of two or more of their tendons to the lower end of the femur, an operation devised by Eggers (1952) for treatment of patients suffering from spastic diplegia. The same objective can be achieved and a weak quadriceps augmented by transfer of the semitendinosus and biceps tendons to the patella.

Foot deformities. These are not only the most common deformities associated with myelomeningocele but often also the most difficult to treat. If full correction cannot be achieved by soft tissue operations at 18–24 months, it is necessary to resort to osteotomy, since inadequate correction is a recipe for pressure sores.

Inversion (varus) deformity is usually due to an unopposed tibialis anterior. In the child with a Type I lesion and motor level of L4, there is usually calcaneovarus; in a Type II lesion, however, equinovarus is likely to result from spasticity of tibialis posterior and calf muscles. Extensive medial release operation is usually required before the foot can be brought into a neutral position. This entails division of not only tibialis anterior but of all tight tendons and ligaments on the medial side of the ankle, with the addition of the tendo Achillis if there is an element of equinus. An attempt can then be made to redistribute active muscles around the ankle, e.g. the tibialis anterior tendon may be transferred to the region of the cuboid bone to supplement weak peronei.

Eversion (valgus) deformity, i.e. the convex boat-shaped foot with vertical talus, is less common but still more difficult to treat. Even the complex procedures described by Sharrard and Grosfield (1968) are liable to be followed by relapse.

Calcaneus deformity is the hallmark of the L5 motor level at which strong dorsiflexors are opposed by paralyzed calf muscles. Without correction, the child will walk on the point of the heel and the forefoot may not touch the ground. Correction is achieved by elongation of the dorsiflexor tendons and maintained by insertion of the tibialis anterior tendon through the interosseous membrane into the heel cord, which provides some plantarflexor power.

Equinus contracture which is due to spasticity of calf muscles is liable to recur after simple section of the tendo Achillis. A more effective procedure is elongation of the tendon which reduces its mechanical advantage. It then is split lengthwise and one half inserted into the dorsum of the foot to augment weak dorsiflexors.

Bracing

With a limited number of active muscles, it may be impossible to achieve complete balance at every joint. Artificial support is then required to maintain the position of function. Strach (1972) has attempted to provide additional 'muscles' by implantation of stainless steel springs in the lower limbs. Technical problems are, however, considerable and success-

Chapter 18

Care at Home

The problems which most worry doctors may differ greatly from those which loom largest for the parents of a child with spina bifida. While their medical advisors are earnestly discussing the child's hydronephrosis or subluxating hip, his father may be struggling to carry him with all his orthopaedic ironmongery up three flights of stairs and his mother engaged in a forlorn attempt to dry countless nappies in a Scottish winter. The two sets of problems are equally real. In comparison, however, to the time and resources expended on the child's medical and surgical treatment, the amount of help given to parents at home is negligible. As noted in Chapter 7, surveys of families with spina bifida children all too often reveal bewildered parents, lacking information, practical and emotional support, who have been left to find their own solution to overwhelming problems which they may not have mentioned in the busy hospital clinic. Although the paediatrician himself may be able to do little he should be able to identify what parents regard as their greatest problems and to recruit whatever assistance they require.

Practical Help

An occupational therapist and social worker visiting the child's home can perhaps best assess the parents' needs for help in dealing with the impact of their child's handicap on everyday life. Furthermore, the advice and guidance they offer at home where mother and child are at ease is more likely to be effective than in hospital where they are often anxious and defensive. Help may be needed in several areas.

Housing. The therapist's suggestions on ways of increasing the child's independence in activities of daily living, such as feeding, dressing, toileting and play, may be difficult to carry out in unsuitable housing conditions. Woodburn (1974) found that two-thirds of affected families were living in unsuitable conditions in South-east Scotland. External and internal stairs are a common hindrance which may make the

136

lavatory inaccessible for the child. Other common problems are doors and passages which are too narrow for a wheelchair, and lack of storage space for all the child's apparatus. Unsuitable housing not only limits the child's independence but increases the mother's work in looking after him. For many families, therefore, nothing can be more helpful than modification of the house or even rehousing. Useful modifications of the house include installation of a ramp to the front door, a low bath, a washing machine or a telephone for parents who may need urgent medical assistance. If the severely handicapped child is unable to go upstairs, the possibility should be considered of extending the house to provide a downstairs toilet and bedroom with additional storage space. In many cases, including the family who lives in a high flat, rehousing on the ground floor with a garden is a simpler solution. If rehousing is necessary, it should if possible be in an area where parents can continue to enjoy support from relatives and friends.

If a medical recommendation accompanies detailed reports on the family's needs from the social worker and occupational therapist, Local Authority Departments are usually sympathetic and constructive in their response. If assistance from other sources is unobtainable the Family Fund may be able to contribute to the cost of approved housing modifications.

Transport. Mobilization of the child has been considered in detail. The mobility of the whole family, so often reduced by the child's handicap, also needs attention. Foster (1973) has shown that the frequency of hospital visiting is inversely related to the distance parents live from the regional paediatric unit. Out-patient clinic attendance is also more difficult for families from remote areas with inadequate public transport. A family car can not only reduce these difficulties but widen the social horizons of the whole family. In appropriate cases, the Family Fund can make a grant for purchase of a car and even for driving lessons.

Recreation. Spina bifida children can often compete on equal terms in traditional paraplegic activities such as archery and table tennis. Swimming and riding can be enjoyed even by more severly handicapped children in special groups arranged by therapists and voluntary organizations such as 'Riding for the Disabled'. Hobbies and other interests encouraged in childhood can contribute to enjoyment of leisure time which may be all too abundant in adult life.

The exceptional difficulties of taking a handicapped child on holiday are recognized by the parents' associations, which provide suitable caravans and holiday homes for the use of members, at modest cost. The Family Fund can also help with the expense of taking a severely handicapped child on holiday. If parents badly need a rest from the care of a child with severe disability, he can usually be admitted to hospital or cared for in one of the excellent holiday homes run by charitable organizations. If relatives are not available to help, shorter periods of relief for parents can be ensured through the babysitting service arranged in most areas by parents' associations.

Financial Assistance

As already indicated, Social Work Departments and the Family Fund are able to give material or financial help for specific purposes. Many children's hospitals have endowment funds which can be used to help parents with items such as the cost of hospital visiting or of replacing clothing devastated by the child's calipers or incontinence.

In addition, however, many parents of spina bifida children in the U.K. are entitled to the Attendance Allowance, a weekly financial allowance from the State. This and other sources of help should be brought to the attention of eligible parents who may be unaware of their existence or reluctant to apply for what they may wrongly construe as 'charity'.

Information

Lack of understanding of their child's problems and treatment is one of the complaints most commonly made by parents. The importance of doctors and nurses giving a clear explanation at every stage of treatment has already been emphasized. The excellent handbooks published by the Spina Bifida Associations should not be regarded as a substitute for direct explanation but as a source of background information to which parents may refer at any time. The publications of the National Children's Bureau which are concerned not with medical and surgical problems but with day-to-day aspects of care and education of the handicapped child can be particularly recommended for parents.

The Spina Bifida Associations not only provide a forum for discussion of parents' problems and for exchange of information but circulate newsletters and supply information on local activities and facilities. Publications which may be of interest to parents (and also to social workers and therapists) are listed at the end of this chapter along with sources of information about services and aids for the handicapped child and his family.

Emotional Support

The need of parents for understanding and emotional support immediately after their child's birth has been emphasized in Chapter 11. When these early crises have been replaced by the long-term prospect of caring for a handicapped child, parents should still have someone to whom they can express their feelings of fear, hostility, frustration and even rejection and from whom they can expect continuing support and reassurance. For many parents who have difficulty in expressing their feelings to one another or to hospital doctors directly involved in their child's treatment, the social worker, health visitor and family doctor can best meet this need. Some parents welcome involvement in the kind of group meetings guided by a social worker which have been described by Linder (1970) and Field (1972).

Counselling is required not only for parents. Siblings whose lives may be overshadowed by the demands of the handicapped child need particular understanding if serious emotional disturbance is to be avoided. Not least, the patient himself may have unexpressed fears and anxieties about his condition and his place in society. He will usually welcome an opportunity of discussing these feelings and obtaining reassurance from the paediatrician or social worker. Patients with more serious difficulties in adjusting to their handicap can benefit from contact with a child psychiatrist. This is most likely to be required in adolescence when the paramount need to conform heightens the handicapped child's awareness of the ways in which he differs from his contemporaries. A group entitled SPOD (Sexual Problems of the Disabled) has recently been set up by the National Fund for Research into Crippling Diseases to study and provide guidance on this difficult and easily neglected aspect of management of the young person with spina bifida.

Sources of Information

Scottish Spina Bifida Association, 7 South East Circus Place, Edinburgh.

Association for Spina Bifida and Hydrocephalus, 30 Devonshire Street, London W1N 2EB.

Disabled Living Foundation, Information Service for the Disabled, 346 Kensington High Street, London W14.

Scottish Council of Social Service, Information Service for the Disabled, 18/19 Claremont Crescent, Edinburgh.

The Family Fund, Joseph Rowntree Memorial Trust, Beverley House, Shipton Road, York YO3 6RB.

British Council for Rehabilitation of the Disabled, Tavistock House, Tavistock Square, London WC1.

Riding for the Disabled, National Equestrian Centre, Kenilworth, Warwickshire.

National Fund for Research into Crippling Diseases, Vincent House, Springfield Road, Horsham, Sussex.

Publications for Parents

The following are published by and obtainable from:

Association for Spina Bifida and Hydrocephalus
Your Child with Spina Bifida   J. Lorber

Day school for the mentally handicapped. Even with a selective approach and optimal treatment, a small but significant proportion of patients will require special education because of mental handicap. Parents who usually have greater difficulty in accepting their child's mental than physical handicap require patient explanation and reassurance when placing the child in this kind of school is recommended.

Residential school. Since Nash, in 1956, emphasized the advantages of a residential special school, there has been a steady trend away from such institutions. They remain of value, however, for the unfortunate minority of patients who come from deprived or broken homes or live in sparsely populated areas without suitable day schools. If residential schooling is necessary, the child should be placed as near to his home and usual treatment centre as possible. In this way, problems of communication between school doctors, nurses and therapists and those who will be responsible for his care during holidays can be minimized.

Temporary provision. Although unsatisfactory on a long-term basis, the hospital school or home teaching can ensure continuation of the child's education during periods of protracted orthopaedic treatment such as spinal fusion.

School Leaving

Even if his schooling has included training in personal independence and social behaviour, school leaving is a major transition for the handicapped child. Aptitude tests as described by Parsons (1972) may be of value in suggesting the types of occupations which are best suited to his talents. Well in advance of the leaving date, a case conference should be held to discuss the child's abilities and weaknesses and to plan for his future. Those involved should include the headmaster, educational psychologist, school medical officer, careers officer, the social worker who will maintain contact when he leaves school and, not least, the parents. The main issues to be discussed will be the possibilities of further education, vocational training and employment.

Few children who have received modern comprehensive treatment for myelomeningocele and hydrocephalus have yet reached school leaving age. The limited information available and experience of other groups of handicapped school leavers suggest, however, that many will have serious difficulty in obtaining employment. There is a need not only for more widespread provision of sheltered workshops with associated hostels, but for more extended education for the handicapped, including vocational training that may prepare them for open employment. It is regrettable that the school leaving age, recently raised for normal children in the U.K., has not been changed for the handicapped who have more than most to gain from a longer stay at school. Furthermore, although 50 per cent of normal children now go on to some kind of further education, only 10 per cent of handicapped school leavers do so (Tuckey *et al.,* 1973). Intensive, and expensive, medical and surgical treatment of children with spina bifida must, if it is to be justified, be matched by opportunities for education and employment which will ensure maximal independence in adult life.

PART 4

MENINGOCELE, SPINA BIFIDA OCCULTA AND RELATED LESIONS

Chapter 20

Simple Meningocele

Clinical Features

As defined in Chapter 2, the simple meningocele contains no neural elements and is associated with no neurological disorder in lower limbs, bladder or bowel. It amounts to no more than a cystic swelling in the thoracic or, more commonly, lumbosacral region which is covered with skin, although this may be thin, pigmented or haemangiomatous. The lesion, containing only CSF, transilluminates freely.

Without surgical exploration, it cannot be distinguished with certainty from a closed myelomeningocele, without apparent neurological involvement. Tenuous skin cover with denuded areas is suggestive of the latter diagnosis, which is confirmed if there is a perineal or lower limb response to faradic stimulation, indicating the presence of nerve roots in the sac. The meningocele must also be differentiated from the skin-covered lipoma with which it may be associated (p. 152).

Associated malformations of the brainstem, axial skeleton and viscera are rare in comparison with their incidence in children suffering from myelomeningocele. Nevertheless, Doran and Guthkelch (1961) reported at least temporarily increased intracranial pressure in 10 per cent, and Milhorat (1972) described associated hydrocephalus due to the Arnold-Chiari malformation in 5 per cent. Experience has shown the incidence of hydrocephalus has been nearer 20 per cent. Ventricular dilatation is seldom gross but the clinical presentation is often acute.

Management

The problem of selection for operation does not arise in infants with simple meningoceles who are unlikely to be appreciably handicapped. Furthermore, as there is no immediate danger of infection or neurological deterioration, surgical intervention is not a matter of urgency. There is, however, no virtue in delaying operation beyond the first few days of life and much to be gained by early repair and discharge home without a worrying lump on the child's back.

Excision of a meningocele is a simple procedure. Since, however, the apparently simple lesion may contain nerve roots and prove to be a closed myelomeningocele or be associated with the intraspinal lesions of 'occult spinal dysraphism' described in Chapter 2, careful exploration of the lesion and underlying theca are mandatory. For this reason, the repair should, if possible, be carried out by a paediatric neurosurgeon.

Follow-up

There is no need for routine air studies or investigation of the urinary tract. Paediatric follow-up is, however, essential in the first 1–2 years. In the early months attention is paid to the head circumference and early signs of hydrocephalus. Later the recognition of minor neurological dysfunction should prompt myelography and urinary tract assessment.

Prognosis

The prognosis is excellent for the child with an uncomplicated meningocele. Since, however, there is an increased risk of more serious neural tube defects in siblings, genetic counselling is indicated, as for the parents of a child with myelomeningocele.

Chapter 21

Spina Bifida Occulta

As noted in Chapter 3, spina bifida occulta is very common and in the vast majority of cases never reaches medical attention. In the minority, it may do so for a wide variety of reasons.

Clinical Presentation

1. Incidental radiological finding. The chance finding of spina bifida occulta, e.g. on IVP films, is frequent and of very little consequence. If the defect is limited to L5 or S1, i.e. is probably a normal variant, and there is no other abnormality, it is very unlikely to be related in any way to nocturnal enuresis, which may have prompted the radiological investigation.

2. Superficial back lesion (Fig. 21.1). The presence of spina bifida occulta may first be suggested by the finding of a cutaneous or other

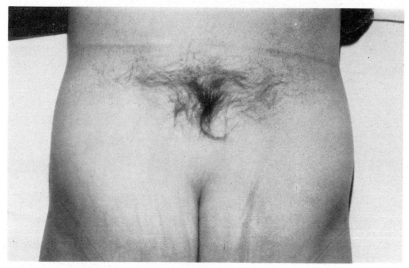

FIG. 21.1. Superficial stigmata of occult spinal dysraphism. (a) Hairy patch.

151

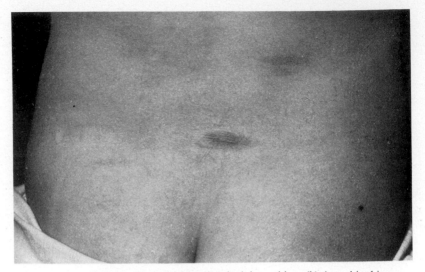

FIG. 21.1. Superficial stigmata of occult spinal dysraphism. (b) Atrophic skin.

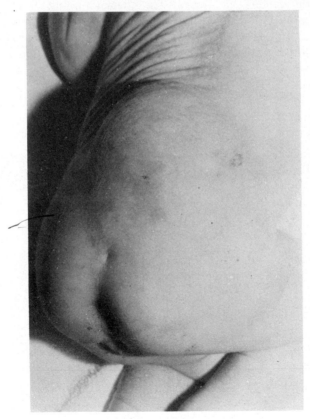

FIG. 21.1. Superficial stigmata of occult spinal dysraphism. (c) Lipoma.

abnormality in the midline of the back. Perhaps the most common is a *tuft of hair* which may be sparse and fine or thick and luxuriant. There may be a *capillary haemangioma* or a *patch of thin, atrophic skin.* A soft, subcutaneous *lipoma* in the sacral region must be differentiated from a skin-covered meningocele. The lipoma is usually flatter, softer, less well-defined than, and more likely than, a meningocele to have normal skin cover. Other common stigmata are skin *dimples* and *bony prominences.*

A midline deffect in the vertebral spines can usually be palpated beneath these cutaneous lesions.

3. Meningitis. A dermal sinus in the lumbar region may first attract attention when it becomes infected or complicated by coliform meningitis. Although it may be marked by a few protruding hairs or a small haemangioma, the opening of a dermal sinus may be very inconspicuous. Such lesions should, therefore, be carefully sought in every child with Gram-negative meningitis and not only when it is recurrent. Chemical meningitis may occur from discharge of cholesterol or sebaceous material from a dermoid cyst into the subarachnoid space. In such cases, sterile CSF (with an excess of polymorphonuclear leucocytes) is found in association with classical signs of meningitis. The glucose level in spinal fluid is normal but cholesterol increased and crystals may be seen on microscopy.

4. Neurological symptoms. A minority of children with the superficial lesions described above present with a neurological syndrome. The pathological varieties of occult spinal dysraphism described in Chapter 2 can interfere with the spinal cord and nerve roots in several ways.

James and Lassman (1962) have emphasized the importance of *traction* on a spinal cord which is tethered and thereby prevented from upward migration in the spinal canal in early childhood. Since it has been shown by Barson (1970b) and others that ascent of the spinal cord is completed in the early months of life, it is more likely, however, that damaging traction on the tethered cord occurs during spinal movement (Guthkelch, 1974). The cause of tethering may be the stalk of a lipoma, a fibrous band or the bony or cartilaginous spur associated with diastematomyelia.

The cord and cauda equina may also be damaged by *direct pressure* from a dermoid cyst, the intraspinal component of a lipoma or a sacral extradural cyst. In some patients, however, the neurological deficit appears to bc due less to an extrinsic lesion than to primary malformation of the cord, i.e. *myelodysplasia,* which may affect only one-half of a split cord.

The neurological syndrome, whatever its cause, is usually milder, slower to develop and less clearly defined than that of myelomeningocele. Unlike open myelomeningocele which is essentially a cord lesion, occult spinal dysraphism may involve nerve roots. It may cause either an upper or lower motor neurone lesion and be reflected by dysfunction of the lower limbs, bladder or both.

If there is *lower limb involvement*, the child usually presents with a limp or foot deformity between the second and fifth year. Examination may reveal a definite neurological abnormality that is commonly asymmetrical. The commoner signs of upper motor neurone involvement are calf spasticity, ankle clonus, extensor plantar responses and an equinovarus deformity. Manifestations of a lower motor neurone lesion include loss of the ankle jerks, pes cavus and clawing of the toes from denervation of foot intrinsic muscles. There may, however, be only a slight asymmetry of gait with turning in of one foot and no definite weakness or wasting on neurological examination. In others, there may be no more than slight underdevelopment of one leg and foot, which may be colder than the other (Fig. 21.2).

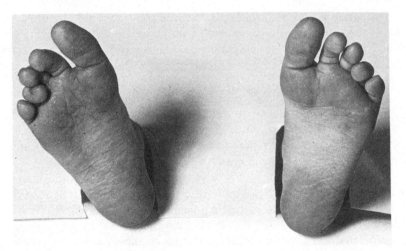

Fig. 21.2. Underdevelopment of left foot due to asymmetrical myelodysplasia (same patient as Fig. 21.1b).

Although motor symptoms usually predominate, they may be accompanied by poorly-defined sensory loss in sacral territory and by vasomotor involvement. Occasionally, the presenting feature is trophic ulceration of the toes due to a combination of arteriolar spasm and anaesthesia (Fig. 21.3).

Despite the mother's insistence that the child is getting worse, it may be difficult for the clinician to decide whether he is dealing with a progressive neurological disorder or purely functional deterioration due to

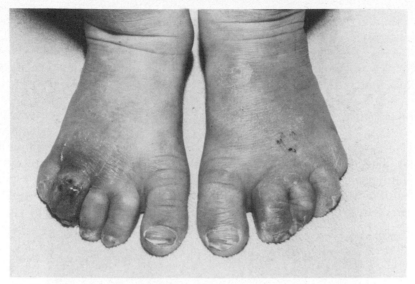

FIG. 21.3. Trophic ulceration of toes (thoracic occult spinal dysraphism).

the child's increasing growth and activity. Rarely symptoms develop in later childhood or even adult life, confirming that restriction of cord migration is not the only cause of damage.

Diastematomyelia is suggested by an asymmetrical neurological deficit and sacral extradural cysts are characterized by late onset of low back pain and sciatica in middle age (Crellin and Jones, 1973). Otherwise, the clinical picture may contain few clues to the exact nature of the lesion involved.

As occult spinal dysraphism usually involves the sacral cord or nerve roots, a *neurogenic bladder* is frequently encountered. If there is weakness of muscles innervated by S2–4 in the legs, some degree of bladder involvement should be expected. Dribbling incontinence of urine may, however, occur before any abnormality of gait and in the absence of any neurological signs in the lower limbs. The types of bladder disorder, the danger of infection and the threat to the upper urinary tract are similar to those already described for myelomeningocele (Hjälmås and Wessner, 1974).

Tragic cases regularly occur of dribbling incontinence due to occult spinal dysraphism in children who have for years been treated for simple enuresis. Before this diagnosis is made, the child should always be examined carefully for a tell-tale lesion on the back, asymmetry of lower limbs or neurological abnormality in S2–4 territory. Conversely, true nocturnal enuresis in which the child may be perfectly dry by day and have occasional dry nights should not be attributed to spina bifida occulta.

Even in patients with urinary incontinence, bowel dysfunction is exceptional.

Associated skeletal malformations are less common than in spina bifida cystica, and hydrocephalus due to the Arnold-Chiari malformation does not occur.

Investigation

Plain x-ray of the spine is indicated in every case and, indeed, without it the diagnosis of spina bifida occulta cannot be made with certainty. Nothing more than the neural arch defect may be seen, but other features which should be looked for (as they are more likely to be associated with a neurological lesion) are widening of the spinal canal, a

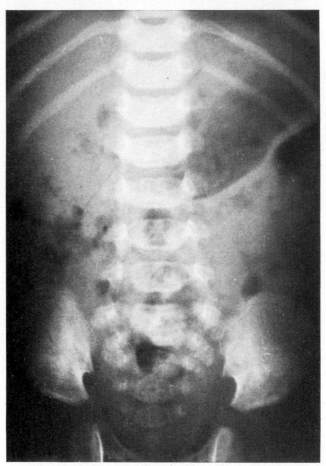

FIG. 21.4. Diastematomyelia. (a) Plain x-ray showing widening of spinal canal at lumbosacral junction and midline spur of bone at S1.

narrow disc space, a mid-line spur of bone or other vertebral anomaly (Fig. 21.4). If spina bifida occulta is limited to the L5 or S1 neural arch and there are no symptoms or signs referable to the lower limbs or bladder, no further investigation is required. If there is an associated cutaneous lesion, careful follow-up is advisable in the first few years of life.

Indications for further investigation include the following:
(a) a more extensive anomaly on plain films of the spine,
(b) asymmetry, deformity or neurological abnormality of the lower limbs, and
(c) urinary incontinence or recurrent urinary infection.

Myelography is the essential investigation in children with any of these criteria. Till (1969) has advocated cisternal myelography in view of the potential danger of lumbar myelography in patients who may have an abnormally low conus medullaris. In the author's experience, however, lumbar myelography has proved to be both safe and satisfactory. Conventional positive contrast examination with Myodil with films taken in both prone and supine position will reveal widening or deformity of the theca and filling defects due to bony or cartilaginous spurs, or to lipomata (Fig. 21.5). These have been well illustrated by Gryspeerdt (1963). The dense Myodil column may, however, fail to demonstrate abnormal tethering of the cord by fibrous bands. For this reason, air myelography may also be of value.

Other investigations such as electromyography and bladder pressure studies may be required to clarify the neurological picture and provide a base-line from which to assess later progress or deterioration.

Differential Diagnosis

In contrast to spina bifida cystica, differential diagnosis may present real problems in spina bifida occulta. If neurological signs or deformity in the lower limbs are attributed uncritically to spina bifida occulta which amounts to no more than a localized vertebral arch defect on x-ray, myelography may be carried out unnecessarily before the correct diagnosis is made.

Spinal tumor, primary or secondary, and *acute myelitis* usually present with rapidly progressive paraplegia and are unlikely to be confused with occult spinal dysraphism in which the history and clinical features, such as lower limb dwarfing or foot deformity, will usually suggest a long-standing lesion.

Greater difficulty may, however, be experienced in differentiating occult spinal dysraphism from other congenital anomalies or familial neurological disorders characterized by foot deformity and/or localized limb weakness. *Peroneal muscular atrophy*, for example, is a chronic

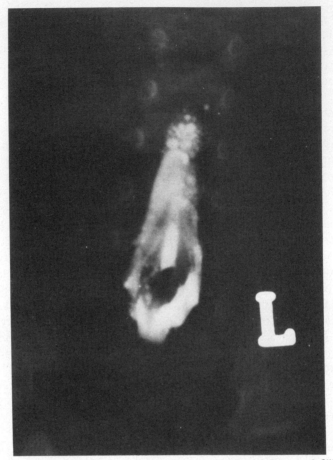

FIG. 21.5. (b) Lumber myelogram showing widening of theca and filling
defect at level of spur.

neuropathy usually inherited as an autosomal dominant and readily
diagnosed in adults by striking distal wasting and weakness in the limbs
accompanied by impairment of reflexes and sensation. In childhood,
however, it may produce little more than pes cavus that is bilateral but
not necessarily symmetrical. The diagnosis is strengthened by a positive
family history of pes cavus and lower limb weakness and can usually be
confirmed by electromyography, which reveals early signs of denervation in peronei and foot intrinsic muscles, and measurement of nerve
conduction velocity, which is reduced at an early stage.

Simple pes cavus, a commoner condition, is also inherited as an autosomal dominant. A positive family history (that may come to light only
with exposure of the parental feet) is against occult spinal dysraphism,
and the finding of normal nerve conduction velocity against a diagnosis
of peroneal muscular atrophy. If, however, the family history is negative,

careful follow-up and/or further investigation are indicated, as already described.

The *hereditary ataxias* are a group of more serious, progressive, familial disorders, the hallmark of which is degeneration of long spinal tracts – pyramidal, posterior columns, spinocerebellar – in various combinations. In childhood, the first feature of familial spastic paraplegia, spinocerebellar degeneration and Friedreich's ataxia is commonly a cavus or cavovarus foot deformity. Careful examination will, however, usually reveal signs of a long tract lesion such as lower limb spasticity or Babinski response, impairment of position and vibration sensation or features of cerebellar ataxia, such as nystagmus and intention tremor.

Not infrequently, a child suffering from a *mild congenital hemiplegia* will present with slight dwarfing, spasticity and equinovarus deformity of one leg, features which may suggest a lesion such as diastematomyelia. Upper limb involvement may be inconspicuous but can usually be demonstrated on careful neurological examination. There may, for example, be asymmetry of associated movements in the arms when the child is asked to walk on his heels or on the lateral edges of his feet; the affected arm may adopt a definitely hemiplegic position when he runs. The diagnosis may also be clinched by detection of a mild facial paresis.

In any of these situations of diagnostic difficulty, a history of incontinence and the finding of dribbling of urine on suprapubic pressure make the diagnosis of occult spinal dysraphism much more likely and myelography mandatory.

Management

The wide spectrum of lesions encompassed by spina bifida occulta is reflected in treatment which ranges from simple reassurance to difficult neurosurgical operation. Management of spina bifida occulta will be considered under the headings of the clinical problems presented.

Isolated radiological defect. Minor degrees of spina bifida occulta discovered incidentally on x-ray require neither further investigation nor treatment.

Cutaneous lesion. A deep or discharging dermal sinus should be excised in view of the risk of abscess formation and meningitis. Such lesions must be carefully traced down to the theca and any associated dermoid cyst removed. If a tuft of hair is causing embarrassment or being caught up in clothing, parents can be reassured that occasional shaving is a harmless solution.

Intraspinal lesion. If myelography reveals an intraspinal lesion laminectomy is indicated. Lesions such as dermoid or extradural cysts can readily be excised. Tethering of the cord can be relieved by resection of bony or cartilaginous spurs or by division of abnormal fibrous attachments. In the case of fibro-lipomatous masses traversed by cauda equina roots, complete excision is dangerous and the neurosurgeon must usually be content to reduce the size of the mass and decompress the neural tissue by extensive laminectomy. Details of surgical technique are recorded in the papers of James and Lassman (1962), Dubowitz *et al.* (1965), Till (1969) and Crellin and Jones (1973).

Neurological sequelae. Following operation, there may be some reduction in the neurological deficit in the lower limbs but incontinence seldom recovers (James and Lassman, 1967). The main aim of operation is, however, to prevent further deterioration and this must be made clear to parents before it is undertaken. Patients who have residual weakness or deformity in the lower limbs or problems associated with neurogenic bladder should be managed in the same way as the child with a myelomeningocele.

Chapter 22

Related Lesions

There remains a miscellaneous group of spinal malformations which embryologically or clinically have features in common with the more familiar lesions already described. Although rare, they will be considered briefly in the interests of completeness.

Anterior Spina Bifida

This term is applied to defects in the vertebral bodies through which the coverings of the spinal cord may protrude or, as described in Chapter 2, communicate with derivatives of the yolk sac. The thoracic, abdominal and pelvic lesions associated with anterior spina bifida are less conspicuous than their posterior counterparts and more varied in their clinical presentation.

Anterior Sacral Meningocele

This lesion protrudes through a well-defined oval defect in the midline or on one side of the sacrum. Like other defects of the caudal cell mass, it may be associated with anorectal malformations. In some cases it is familial with autosomal or sex-linked dominant inheritance (Klenerman and Merrick, 1973; Cohn and Bay-Nielsen, 1969).

The condition seldom presents in infancy unless it is discovered by chance on radiological examination. If it declares itself in childhood it is usually with symptoms of pelvic obstruction such as constipation, dysuria or urinary retention. Less frequently still, there are features of nerve root involvement such as incontinence, paralysis and sensory loss in sacral territory. Later in life, it may present to the obstetrician as an 'ovarian cyst' or to the surgeon as an acute abdomen. In these situations, puncture or incision of the lesion in ignorance of its nature may be followed by meningitis.

The meningocele may be palpable on rectal examination and radiological examination will usually establish its origin. If the sacral defect is lateral, the intact half of the sacrum is seen to curve round the margin of the lesion in a 'sickle' shape. Midline defects are less obvious on anteroposterior projections, but lateral films show the tip of the sacrum and coccyx curving forwards below the mass. While myelography usually delineates the meningeal sac, it may be negative if the communication with the spinal theca is very narrow.

Although some advocate an expectant approach if the patient is asymptomatic, Thierry *et al.* (1969), on the basis of an extensive review of the literature, advocate resection in view of the risks of spontaneous rupture and, in the young female, of later obstetric complications.

Intrathoracic Meningocele

Anterior meningoceles also occur in relation to the thoracic spine and present as mediastinal masses. The majority of affected patients, however, are suffering from von Recklinghausen's disease and have obvious café-au-lait spots and cutaneous neurofibromata. In such cases the bony defect is not in the vertebral bodies but in the pedicles which are softened or eroded by neurofibromatosis (La Vielle and Campbell, 1958).

Neurenteric Cyst

The neurenteric cyst, derived from the yolk sac, is lined with oesophageal, gastric or intestinal mucosa. It is situated in the posterior mediastinum usually in relation to the second thoracic vertebra and is connected to the meninges or spinal cord by a stalk which passes through the anterior vertebral defect.

The early clinical features are usually related to mediastinal compression, e.g. cough and dyspnoea. Chest x-ray prompted by such symptoms reveals the characteristic combination of a circumscribed mediastinal mass and anomalous vertebral development (Fig. 22.1). The neurenteric cyst has, however, an extensive repertoire of symptomatology. Upper limb weakness, e.g. wasting of the small muscles of the hands, and lower limb spasticity can occur if an intrathecal extension of the lesion involves the spinal cord or thoracic nerve roots. Clinical and CSF features of acute pyogenic meningitis have recently been seen from secretion of hydrochloric acid into the theca by a lesion lined with gastric mucosa.

Treatment is surgical removal of the lesion which may be difficult and involve a combination of thoractomy and laminectomy.

Sacral Agenesis

Partial agenesis of the sacrum may, as described, be associated with an anterior meningocele. A more extensive sacral defect may, however,

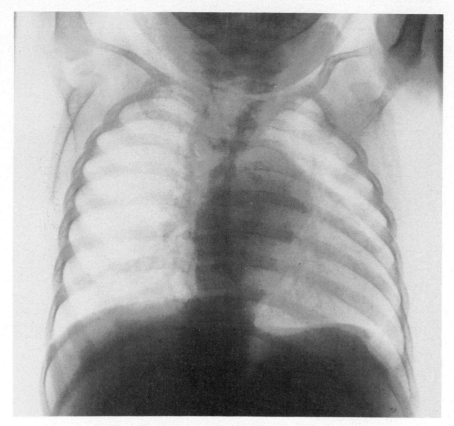

FIG. 22.1. Neurenteric cyst: x-ray showing mediastinal mass and anomalous thoracic vertebrae.

occur which is accompanied by failure of development of related nerve roots. Since Landauer demonstrated in 1945 that sacral agenesis could be induced in fowls by insulin injection, there have been numerous reports of an increased incidence in infants of diabetic mothers. Combining several published series with their own, Banta and Nichols (1969) estimated that 19 per cent of patients with sacral agenesis had insulin-treated diabetic mothers.

Even complete sacral agenesis is not always obvious at birth. There is, however, prominence of the last lumbar vertebra below which the buttocks are abnormally flat (Fig. 22.2). Some degree of paralysis, reflex and sensory loss is usually found in sacral territory and associated with an inert neurogenic bladder. The motor level usually corresponds to the lowest normal vertebral body. Absence of the sacrum is easily confirmed by rectal examination and radiological examination, which also shows an unusually narrow pelvis.

No specific treatment is possible but the orthopaedic and urological

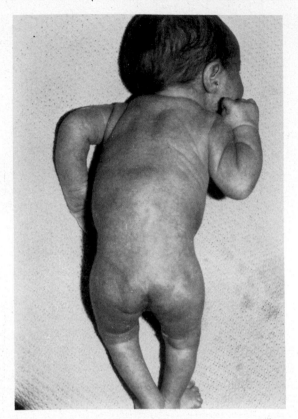

FIG. 22.2. Sacral agenesis. (a) Clinical appearance in infancy.

problems are managed as in the child with a myelomeningocele. Residual disability is greatest in patients who have agenesis not only of the sacrum but of the lower lumbar vertebrae with collapse of the ilio-spinal junction and extensive neurological involvement. Although intertrochanteric amputation has been customary in these patients, Banta and Nichols (1969) have had a measure of success with more conservative correction of deformities and bracing of the lower limbs.

Sacrococcygeal Teratoma

This embryonal tumour contains a variety of tissues including bone and cartilage, intestinal and respiratory epithelium and neural or glial elements. These derivatives of the three germinal layers may be combined to form rudimentary limbs or organs.

It is usually evident at birth as a large skin-covered mass protruding from the sacrococcygeal region in the midline (Fig. 22.3). It may, however, be apparent only on careful examination, as slight fullness

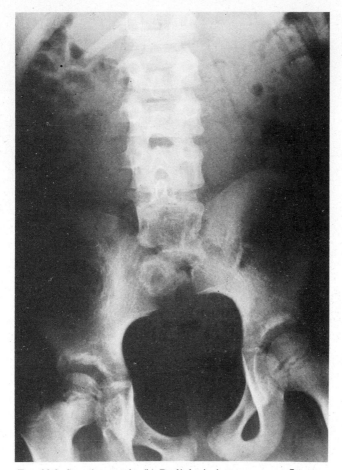

FIG. 22.2. Sacral agenesis. (b) Radiological appearance at 7 years.

or asymmetry of the buttocks or sacral region. An appreciable proportion of patients have other malformations in tissues derived from the caudal cell mass, e.g. anomalies of the sacral vertebrae, anorectum and genito-urinary tract. Neurological involvement is, however, rare.

If early diagnosis is followed by complete excision of the lesion, the prognosis is excellent. If, however, a teratoma is missed in infancy and treatment delayed, there is a high risk of malignant change and wide-spread metastasis (McDonald, 1973).

Cranium Bifidum

Lesions analogous to open myelomeningocele, closed myelomeningocele and simple meningocele occur from anomalous development of the

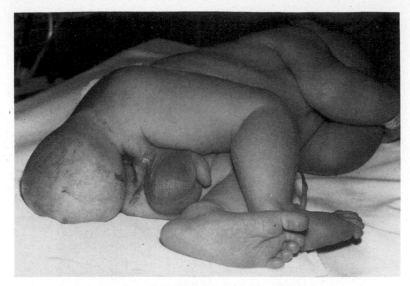

FIG. 22.3. Sacrococcygeal teratoma.

cranial reaches of the neural tube, viz. anencephaly, encephalocele and occipital meningocele. These craniocerebral malformations are, however, beyond the scope of a book on spina bifida.

PART 5

THE FUTURE

Chapter 23

Prevention

Our understanding of the aetiology of spina bifida cystica as outlined in Chapter 3 is still too limited to be of great value in prevention. Until they have produced their first affected child, there is nothing to distinguish parents who are genetically at risk and the important environmental trigger continues to operate incognito. Although true aetiological prevention is no more than a hope for the future, measures now available can achieve a modest reduction in the incidence of spina bifida cystica and offer the prospect of more substantial reduction in the not too distant future. These measures are genetic counselling and antenatal diagnosis.

Genetic Counselling

Genetic counselling should be offered to all parents who have had an infant suffering from either anencephaly or spina bifida cystica. The optimal time is probably within a month of the child's birth but not in the immediate neonatal period when it may do little more than increase their feelings of confusion, guilt and inadequacy. The paediatrician who has already established a rapport with the parents is usually the most appropriate genetic counsellor. If confusion is to be avoided, his message must also be made known to the family doctor and social worker who may be consulted about its implications.

The precise risk of recurrence of a neural tube defect in a sibship depends on the local incidence, but in the U.K. it is of the order of 1 in 20 when one child has been affected and 1 in 8 after the birth of 2 affected children. The occurrence of early miscarriage can, for practical purposes, be ignored but the recurrence risk is increased by consanguinity (Carter, 1974). If the affected child had spina bifida, approximately two-thirds of the risk is for spina bifida and one-third for anencephaly, and vice versa.

The risk of parents having another *handicapped* child is, however, considerably less than the 1 in 20 figure quoted above since it encom-

169

passes the possibility of a stillborn anencephalic child, an infant with extensive myelomeningocele who is unlikely to be selected for operation and the child with a simple meningocele without neurological involvement. The risk of parents having another child who survives the neonatal period with significant disability is, therefore, unlikely to be more than 1 in 50, a less forbidding prospect for parents who are anxious to have another child. If the decision, which must finally be the parents' own, is against having further pregnancies, the paediatrician must ensure that they have access to practical contraceptive help.

The limited evidence so far available suggests that the offspring of adult survivors with spina bifida will have a 3–4 per cent incidence of neural tube defects (Lorber, 1971c; Tünte, 1971). Children of the patient's siblings have a lower risk and those of his aunts and uncles only twice that of the population at large.

Antenatal Diagnosis

In addition to information on the risks of recurrence, parents who have no religious or ethical objections to abortion of an affected fetus can now be offered antenatal diagnosis should they opt for another pregnancy.

Antenatal diagnosis depends on the finding of elevated levels of alpha-fetoprotein (APP), a fetal serum protein, in amniotic fluid surrounding fetuses with anencephaly and open myelomeningocele (Brock and Sutcliffe, 1972). The reliability with which these conditions can be detected by amniocentesis at 14–16 weeks gestation has been confirmed repeatedly since the original report from Edinburgh (*British Medical Journal*, 1975).

The possibility of termination of a second affected pregnancy offers new hope to parents already afflicted. Since, however, few patients are second affected children, antenatal diagnosis of this kind cannot reduce the overall incidence of neural tube defects by much more than 5 per cent. The search has, therefore, already begun for techniques which might be more suitable than amniocentesis, which is not without risk, for routine screening of *all* pregnancies.

The most promising measure at present is estimation of the maternal *serum level* of AFP (Wald *et al.*, 1974; Brock *et al.*, 1974). In contrast to amniotic fluid levels, serum AFP is low in the first trimester and may not reach diagnostically significant levels until the fifth month of gestation. Although not all affected pregnancies will be detected between 14 and 21 weeks, high serum AFP levels justify amniocentesis if multiple pregnancy (another cause of high levels) has been excluded by ultrasonography. Pilot screening programmes of this kind are already being assessed in several centres while the search continues for other fetal proteins which could betray an affected pregnancy.

For many parents and doctors, however, the prospect of accurate antenatal diagnosis is shadowed by ethical problems no less serious than those associated with selective operation in the newborn period. These two unhappy compromises are for the present our best hope of reducing the incidence of spina bifida on the one hand and the survival of grossly handicapped children on the other. A happier solution to the overwhelming problems of spina bifida can, however, emerge only from a clearer understanding of its aetiology.

'. . . the end of all our exploring
Will be to arrive where we started
and know the place for the first time'
T. S. Eliot.

References

ALKER G.J., GLASAVER F.E. & LESLIE E.V. (1973) The radiology of CSF shunts and their complications. *British Journal of Radiology* **46**, 496.

ALLUM N. (1975) *Spina bifida. The treatment and care of spina bifida children.* London: George Allen & Unwin Ltd.

ANDERSON F.M. (1968) Occult spinal dysraphism. *Journal of Pediatrics* **73**, 163.

AREY L.B. (1965) *Developmental anatomy. A textbook and laboratory manual of embryology* 7th Ed. Philadelphia: W.B. Saunders.

ARNEIL G.C., McALLISTER T.A. & KAY P. (1973) Management of bacteriuria by plane dipslide culture. *Lancet* **i**, 94.

BADELL-RIBERA A., SHULMAN K. & PADDOCK N. (1966) The relationship of non-progressive hydrocephalus to intellectual functioning in children with spina bifida cystica. *Pediatrics* **37**, 787.

BAKER R.H. & SHARRARD W.J.W. (1973) Correction of lordoscoliosis in spina bifida by multiple spinal osteotomy and fusion with Dwyer fixation: a preliminary report. *Developmental Medicine and Child Neurology,* Supplement **29**, 12.

BANTA J.V. & NICHOLS O. (1969) Sacral agenesis. *Journal of Bone and Joint Surgery* **51A**, 693.

BARRY A., PATTEN B.M. & STEWART B.H. (1957) Possible factors in development of the Arnold-Chiari malformation. *Journal of Neurosurgery* **14**, 285.

BARSON A.J. (1970a) Spina bifida – the significance of the level and extent of the defect to the morphogenesis. *Developmental Medicine and Child Neurology* **12**, 129.

BARSON A.J. (1970b) The vertebral level of termination of the spinal cord during normal and abnormal development. *Journal of Anatomy* **106**, 489.

BAYSTON R. (1975) Antibiotic prophylaxis in shunt surgery. *Developmental Medicine and Child Neurology,* Supplement **35**, 99.

BAYSTON R. & LARI J. (1974) A study of the sources of infection in colonised shunts. *Developmental Medicine and Child Neurology,* Supplement **32**, 16.

BAYSTON R. & PENNY S.R. (1972) Excessive production of mucoid substance in Staphylococcus SIIA: a possible factor in colonisation of Holter shunts. *Developmental Medicine and Child Neurology,* Supplement **27**, 25.

BECKER D.P. & NULSEN F.E. (1968) Control of hydrocephalus by valve regulated venous shunt. Avoidance of complications in prolonged shunt maintenance. *Journal of Neurosurgery* **28**, 215.

BÉCLARD (1816) cited by Fraser (1929).

BERGSTRÖM T., LINCOLN K., ORSKOV F., ORSKOV I. & WINBERG J. (1967) Studies of urinary tract infections in infancy and childhood. VIII. Reinfection vs. relapse. *Journal of Pediatrics* **71**, 13.

BLAZÉ J.B., FORREST D.M. & TSINGOGLOU S. (1971) Atriotomy using the Holter shunt in hydrocephalus. *Developmental Medicine and Child Neurology,* Supplement **25**, 27.

BLOCKEY N.J. (1971) Aids for crippled children. *Developmental Medicine and Child Neurology* **13**, 216.

BOKINSKY G.E., HUDSON L.D. & WEIL J.V. (1973) Impaired peripheral chemosensitivity and acute respiratory failure in Arnold-Chiari malformation and syringomyelia. *New England Journal of Medicine* **288**, 947.

BRICKER E.M. (1950) Bladder substitution after pelvic evisceration. *Surgical Clinics of North America* **30**, 1511.

BRITISH MEDICAL JOURNAL (1972) Editorial. Diet and congenital defects. *British Medical Journal* **4**, 684.

BRITISH MEDICAL JOURNAL (1975) Antenatal diagnosis of spina bifida. *British Medical Journal* **i**, 414.

BROCK D.J.H., BOLTON A.E. & SCRIMGEOUR J.B. (1974) Prenatal diagnosis of spina bifida and anencephaly through maternal plasma-alpha-fetoprotein measurement. *Lancet* **i**, 767.

BROCK D.J.H. & SUTCLIFFE R.G. (1972) Alpha-fetoprotein in the antenatal diagnosis of anencephaly and spina bifida. *Lancet* **ii**, 197.

BROCKLEHURST G., GLEAVE J.R.D. & LEWIN N. (1966) Early closure of myelomeningocele with especial reference to leg movement. *Developmental Medicine and Child Neurology*, Supplement **13**, 51.

BRISMAN R., STEIN B.M. & JOHNSON P.M. (1970) Lung scan and shunted childhood hydrocephalus. *Developmental Medicine and Child Neurology*, Supplement **22**, 18.

BUCHANAN R. & MULLINS J.B. (1968) Integration of a spina bifida child in a kindergarten for normal children. *Young Children* **23**, 6, 339.

BUTLER N.R. & BONHAM D.G. (1963) *Perinatal Mortality*. Edinburgh: Livingstone.

CALDWELL K.P.S. (1968) The use of electrical stimulation in urinary retention and incontinence. Proceedings of the Royal Society of Medicine, **61**, 703.

CALDWELL K.P.S., FLACK F.C. & BROAD A.F. (1965) Urinary incontinence following spinal injury by electronic implant. *Lancet* **i**, 846.

CALDWELL K.P.S., MARTIN M.R., FLACK F.C. & JAMES E.D. (1969) An alternative method of dealing with incontinence in children with neurogenic bladders. *Archives of Disease in Childhood* **44**, 625.

CARTER C.O. (1974) Clues to the aetiology of neural tube malformations. *Developmental Medicine and Child Neurology*, Supplement **32**, 3.

CARTER C.O. & FRASER ROBERTS J.A. (1967) The risk of recurrence after two children with central nervous system malformations. *Lancet* **i**, 306.

CAVINESS V.S. (1976) The Chiari malformations of the posterior fossa and their relation to hydrocephalus. *Developmental Medicine and Child Neurology* (in press).

CHADD M.A., GRAY O.P. & KEYSER J.W. (1970) Gamma globulin levels in newborn infants with spina bifida cystica. *Acta Paediatrica Scandinavica* **59**, 134.

CHANTRAINE A., LLOYD K. & SWINYARD C.A. (1966) The sphincter ani extremus in spina bifida and myelomeningocele. *Journal of Neurology* **95**, 250.

CHESTER D.C., PENNY S.R. & EMERY J.L. (1971) Fat-containing macrophages in the cerebrospinal fluid of children with hydrocephalus. *Developmental Medicine and Child Neurology*, Supplement **25**, 33.

CHIARI H. (1891) Über Veränderungen des Kleinhirns in folge von Hydrocephalie des Grosschirns. *Deutsch. Med. Wschs.* **17**, 1172.

CLELAND J. (1883) Study of spina bifida, encephalocele and anencephalus. *Journal of Anatomical Physiology* **17**, 257.

COFFEY V.P. & JESSOP W.J. (1957) A study of 137 cases of anencephaly. *British Journal of Preventive and Social Medicine* **11**, 174.

COHN J.C. & BAY-NIELSEN E. (1969) Hereditary defect of sacrum and coccyx with anterior sacral meningocele. *Acta Paediatrica Scandinavica* **58**, 268.

COLLIS V.R. (1972) The effects of selective treatment on a neonatal unit. *Developmental Medicine and Child Neurology*, Supplement **27**, 34.

COOK R.C.M., LISTER J. & ZACHARY R.B. (1968) Operative management of the neurogenic bladder in children – diversion through ileal conduits. *Surgery* **63**, 825.

COOPER D.G.W. (1967) Urinary tract infection in children with myelomeningocele. *Archives of Disease in Childhood* **42**, 521.

COOPER D.G.W. (1968) Detrusor action in children with myelomeningocele. *Archives of Disease in Childhood* **43**, 427.

CRELLIN R.Q. & JONES E.R. (1973) Sacral Extradural Cysts: a rare cause of low backache and sciatica. *Journal of Bone and Joint Surgery* **55B**, 20.

CUDMORE R.E. & ZACHARY R.B. (1970) The renogram and the renal tract in spina bifida. *Developmental Medicine and Child Neurology*, Supplement **22**, 24.

CUENDET A. (1969) Le problème de la fonction, ano-rectale dans la myéloméningocèle. *Annales de Chirurgie Infantile (Paris)* **10**, 81.

CURTIS B.H. & FISHER R.L. (1969) Congenital hyperextension with anterior subluxation of the knee. Surgical treatment and long-term observations. *Journal of Bone and Joint Surgery* **51A**, 258.

CZEIZEL A. & REVESZ C. (1970) Major malformations of the nervous system in Hungary. *British Journal of Preventive and Social Medicine* **24**, 205.

D'ARCY E. (1968) Congenital Defects: Mother's first reaction to information. *British Medical Journal* **iii**, 796.

DARESTI (1877) Production artificielle des monstruosités. Cited by Fraser, J. (1929).

DE LANGE S.A. (1974) Selection in the management of patients with spina bifida aperta. *Developmental Medicine and Child Neurology*, Supplement **32**, 27.

DICKSON J.A.S. (1975) Personal communication.

DICKSON J.A.S., ECKSTEIN H.B., GLASSON M.J. & KAPKA L. (1968) Shunt surgery in hydrocephalus after blockage of both internal jugular veins. *Developmental Medicine and Child Neurology*, Supplement **16**, 110.

DICKSON J.A.S. & NIXON H.H. (1968) Control by electronic stimulator of incontinence after operation for anorectal atresia. *Journal of Pediatric Surgery* **3**, 696.

DORAN P.A. & GUTHKELCH A.N. (1961) Studies in spina bifida cystica. Part 1: General survey and reassessment of the problem. *Journal of Neurology, Neurosurgery and Psychiatry* **24**, 331.

DORFF G.B. & SHAPIRO L.M. (1937) Clinicopathologic study of sexual precocity with hydrocephalus: report of two cases occurring in females with post mortem observations in one. *Americal Journal of Diseases of Childhood* **53**, 481.

DORNER S. (1973) Psychological and social problems of families of adolescent spina bifida patients: a preliminary report. *Developmental Medicine and Child Neurology*, Supplement **29**, 24.

DRENNAN J.C. (1970) The role of muscles in the development of human lumbar kyphosis. *Developmental Medicine and Child Neurology*, Supplement **22**, 33.

DRUMMOND M.B. & BELTON N.R. (1972) Creatine phospho-kinase in the CSF: its value in the management of children with myelomeningocele and hydrocephalus. *Archives of Disease in Childhood* **47**, 672.

DRUMMOND M.B. & DONALDSON A.A. (1974) Air, Myodil and Conray studies in the hydrocephalus of myelomeningocele. *Developmental Medicine and Child Neurology*, Supplement **32**, 131.

DUBOWITZ V., LORBER J. & ZACHARY R.B. (1965) Lipoma of the cauda equina. *Archives of Disease in Childhood* **40**, 207.

DUCKWORTH T., SHARRARD W.J.W., LISTER J. & SEYMOUR N. (1968) Hemimyelocele. *Developmental Medicine and Child Neurology*, Supplement **16**, 191.

DUHAMEL B. (1969) In discussion of paper by Cuendet (1969). *Annales de Chirurgie Infantile* (Paris) **10**, 86.

DUNSDON M.I. (1953) Comparison of Terman Merrill scale test responses among large-scale samples of normal, maladjusted and backward children. *Journal of Mental Sciences* **99**, 720.

DUTHIE E.J.W. & STARK G.D. (1974) Catheters for Continence. A preliminary report on their trial in myelomeningocele. *Developmental Medicine and Child Neurology*, Supplement **32**, 31.

DWYER A.F., NEWTON N.C. & SHERWOOD A.A. (1969) An anterior approach to scoliosis. *Clinical Orthopaedics and Related Research* **62**, 192.

ECKSTEIN H.B. (1968) Urinary control in children with myelomeningocele. *British Journal of Urology* **40**, 191.

ECKSTEIN H.B. (1974) The treatment of the neuropathic bladder by transmitted electrical stimulation. *Lancet* **i**, 780.

ECKSTEIN H.B. & MOHINDRA P. (1970) The defunctioned neurogenic bladder: a clinical study. *Developmental Medicine and Child Neurology*, Supplement **22**, 46.

EDVARDSEN P. (1972) Physeo-epiphyseal injuries of lower extremities in myelomeningocele. *Acta Orthopaedica Scandinavica* **43**, 550.

EDWARDS J.H. (1958) Congenital malformations of the central nervous system in Scotland. *British Journal of Preventive and Social Medicine* **12**, 115.

EGGERS G.W.N. (1952) Transplantation of hamstring tendons to femoral condyles in order to improve hip extension and to decrease knee flexion in cerebral spastic paralysis. *Journal of Bone and Joint Surgery* **34A**, 827.

ELLIS H.L. (1974) Parental involvement in the decision to treat spina bifida cystica. *British Medical Journal* **i**, 369.

ELWOOD J.H. & NEVIN N.C. (1973) Factors associated with anencephaly and spina bifida in Belfast. *British Journal of Preventive and Social Medicine* **27**, 73.

EMERY J.L. & HILTON H.B. (1961) Lung and heart complications of the treatment of hydrocephalus by ventriculoauriculostomy. *Surgery* **50**, 309.

EMERY J.L. & LENDON R.G. (1969) Lipomas of the cauda equina and other fatty tumours related to neurospinal dysraphism. *Developmental Medicine and Child Neurology*, Supplement **20**, 62.

EMERY J.L. & LENDON R.G. (1973) The local cord lesion in neurospinal dysraphism (meningomyelocele). *Journal of Pathology* **110**, 83.

EMERY J.L. & SVITORK I. (1967) Intrahemispherical distances in congenital hydrocephalus associated with meningomyelocele. *Developmental Medicine and Child Neurology*, Supplement **15**, 21.

EMMETT J.L. & SIMON H.B. (1956) Transurethral resection in infants and children for congenital obstruction of the vesical neck and myelodysplasia. *Journal of Urology* **76**, 595.

EPSTEIN F., HOCHWALD M. & RANSOHOFF J. (1973) Neonatal hydrocephalus treated by compressive head wrapping. *Lancet* **i**, 634.

EPSTEIN F., RUBIN R. & HOCHWALD G.M. (1974) Restoration of the cortical mantle in severe feline hydrocephalus: a new laboratory model. *Developmental Medicine and Child Neurology*, Supplement **32**, 49.

ERICSSON N.O., HELLSTRÖM B., NERGÅRDH A. & RUDHE U. (1970) Unilateral neurological defect in myelomeningocele with normal bladder function. *Acta Paediatrica Scandinavica* **59**, 487.

FEREMBACH D. (1963) Frequency of spina bifida occulta in prehistoric human skeletons. *Nature* **199**, 100.

FIELD B. (1972) The child with spina bifida. Medical and social aspects of the problems of a child with multiple handicaps and his family. *Medical Journal of Australia* **2**, 1284.

FOLTZ E.L. & SHURTLEFF D.B. (1963) Five-year comparative study of hydrocephalus in children with and without operation. *Journal of Neurosurgery* **20**, 1064.

FORREST D.M. (1974) The use of the Foley catheter for long-term urine collection in girls. *Developmental Medicine and Child Neurology*, Supplement **32**, 54.

FORREST D.M. & TSINGOGLOU S. (1968) The false fontanelle as a practical method of long-term testing of intracranial pressure. *Developmental Medicine and Child Neurology*, Supplement **16**, 17.

FORSYTHE W.I. & KINLEY J.G. (1970) Bowel control of children with spina bifida. *Developmental Medicine and Child Neurology* **12**, 27.

FOSTER F. (1973) Ph.D. Thesis (University of Edinburgh).

FRASER J. (1929) Spina bifida. *Edinburgh Medical Journal* **36**, 284.

FREESTON B.M. (1971) An enquiry into the effect of a spina bifida child upon family life. *Developmental Medicine and Child Neurology* **13**, 456.

GARDNER W.J. (1961) Rupture of the neural tube. The cause of myelomeningocele. *Archives of Neurology* **4**, 13.

GIBNEY H. (1970) *Your Child and Ileal Conduit Surgery: a guide book for parents.* Springfield, Ill.: Charles C. Thomas.

GRYSPEERDT G.L. (1963) Myelographic assessment of occult forms of spinal dysraphism. *Acta radiologica* (diagn.) **1**, 702.

GUBBAY S.S. (1966) Derangement of temperature control in hydrocephalus. *Developmental Medicine and Child Neurology*, Supplement **13**, 125.

GUILLAME J. & ROGÉ R. (1950) Troubles neuro-endocriniens et hydrocéphalic chronique. *Revue Neurologique* **82**, 424.

GULLIFORD R. (1975) *Helping the handicapped child. 2. At school.* Windsor: N.F.E.R. Publishing Company Ltd., for National Children's Bureau.

GUTHKELCH A. N. (1974) Diastematomyelia with median septum. *Brain* **97**, 729.

HABIB H.N. (1963) Neural trigger points for evacuation of neurogenic bladder by electro-stimulation. *Surgical Forum* **14**, 489.

HAGBERG B. (1962) The sequelae of spontaneously arrested infantile hydrocephalus. *Developmental Medicine and Child Neurology* **4**, 583.

HAGBERG B. & SJÖGREN I. (1966) The chronic brain syndrome of infantile hydrocephalus. A follow-up study of 63 spontaneously arrested cases. *Americal Journal of Diseases of Children* **112**, 189.

HALEVI H.S. (1967) Congenital malformation in Israel. *British Journal of Preventive and Social Medicine* **21**, 66.

HALVERSTADT D.B. & LEADBETTER W.F. (1968) Electrical stimulation of the human bladder: experience in three patients with hypotonic neurogenic bladder dysfunction. *British Journal of Urology* **40**, 175.

HAMILTON W.J. & MOSSMAN H.W. (1972) *Human Embryology*. 4th Ed. Cambridge: W. Heffer and Sons Ltd.

HARE E.G., LAURENCE K.M., PAYNE H. & RAWNSLEY K. (1966) Spina bifida cystica and family stress. *British Medical Journal* **ii**, 757.

HAY M.C. & WALKER G. (1973) Plantar pressures in healthy children and in children with myelomeningocele. *Journal of Bone and Joint Surgery* **55B**, 828.

HAYDEN P.W., FOLTZ E.L. & SHURTLEFF D.B. (1968) Effect of an oral osmotic agent on ventricular fluid pressure of hydrocephalic children. *Pediatrics* **41**, 955.

HAYES-ALLEN M.C. & TRING F.C. (1973) Obesity: another hazard for spina bifida children. *British Journal of Preventive and Social Medicine* **27**, 192.

HEATLEY C.A. (1939) The larynx in infancy. A study of chronic stridor. *Archives of Otolaryngology* **29**, 90.

HEIMBURGER R.F. (1972) Early repair of myelomeningocele. *Journal of Neurosurgery* **37**, 594.

HERZOG, E.G. & SHARRARD W.J.W. (1966) Calipers and brace with double hip lock. *Clinical Orthopaedics and Related Research* **46**, 239.

HIDE D.W. & SEMPLE C. (1970) Coordinated care of the child with spina bifida. *Lancet* **ii**, 603.

HIDE D.W., WILLIAMS H.P. & ELLIS H.L. (1972) The outlook for the child with a myelo-meningocele for whom early surgery was considered inadvisable. *Developmental Medicine and Child Neurology* **14**, 304.

HJÄLMÅS K. & WESSNER G. (1974) Examination of bladder function in occult spinal dysraphism. *Developmental Medicine and Child Neurology*, Supplement **32**, 156.

HOLT R.J. (1969) The classification of staphylococci from colonised ventriculo-atrial shunts. *Journal of Clinical Pathology* **22**, 475.

HOLT R.J. (1970) Bacteriological studies on colonised ventriculo-atrial shunts. *Developmental Medicine and Child Neurology*, Supplement **22**, 83.

HOPKINSON B.R. & LIGHTWOOD R. (1967) Electrical treatment of incontinence. *British Journal of Surgery* **54**, 802.

HOSKING G.P. (1974) Fits in hydrocephalic children. *Archives of Disease in Childhood* **49**, 633.

HOWAT J.M. (1971) Urinary ascites complicating spina bifida. *Archives of Disease in Childhood* **46**, 103.

HUNT G.M. (1973) Implications of the treatment of myelomeningocele for the child and his family. *Lancet* **ii**, 1308.

HUNT G.M. & HOLMES A.E. (1975) Some factors relating to intelligence in treated cases of spina bifida. *Developmental Medicine and Child Neurology*, Supplement **35**, 65.

HUNT G., LEWIS L., GLEAVE J. & GAIRDNER D. (1973) Predictive factors in open myelo-meningocele with special reference to sensory level. *British Medical Journal* **iv**, 197.

INGRAM T.T.S. (1962a) Congenital ataxic syndromes in cerebral palsy. *Acta Paediatrica (Scand.)* **51**, 209.

INGRAM T.T.S. (1962b) Ataxia and ataxic diplegia in childhood. In *Cerebellum, Posture and Cerebral Palsy*. National Spastics Society Medical Education and Information Unit in association with William Heinemann Medical Books Ltd., London.

INGRAM T.T.S. & NAUGHTON J.A. (1962) Paediatric and psychological aspects of cerebral palsy associated with hydrocephalus. *Developmental Medicine and Child Neurology* **4**, 287.

IRELAND G.W. & GEIST R.W. (1970) Difficulties with vesicostomies in 15 children with myelomeningocele. *Journal of Urology* **103**, 341.

ISAMAT F. (1969) Bronchovenous fistula as a late complication of ventriculo atriostomy. Case report. *Journal of Neurosurgery* **31**, 574.

JAMES C.C.M. (1970) Fractures of the lower limbs in spina bifida cystica: a survey of 44 fractures in 122 children. *Developmental Medicine and Child Neurology,* Supplement **22**, 88.

JAMES C.C.M. & LASSMAN L.P. (1962) Spinal Dysraphism: The diagnosis and treatment of progressive lesions in spina bifida occulta. *Journal of Bone and Joint Surgery* **44B**, 828.

JAMES C.C.M. & LASSMAN L.P. (1967) Results of treatment of progressive lesions in spina bifida occulta 5 to 10 years after laminectomy. *Lancet* **ii**, 1277.

JÉZÉQUEL C., JÉZÉQUEL J., JÉHAN P. & COUTEL Y. (1971) Troubles de la déglutition au cours des spina bifida du nourrisson. *Archives françaises de Pédiatrie* **28**, 901.

JOBLING M. (1975) *Helping the handicapped child. 1. In the family.* Windsor: N.F.E.R. Publishing Co. Ltd., for National Childrens Bureau, London.

JONGE M.C. DE, CORNELIUS J.A. & BERG J.W. VAN DEN (1969) The evaluation of functional disorders of the urinary tract in children with spina bifida. *Developmental Medicine and Child Neurology,* Supplement **20**, 51.

KARLIN I.W. (1935) Incidence of spina bifida occulta in children with and without enuresis. *American Journal of Diseases of Children* **49**, 125.

KATONA F. (1958) Electric stimulation in the diagnosis and therapy of bladder paralysis. *Orvosi Hetilap* **99**, 277.

KATONA F. & ECKSTEIN H.B. (1974) Treatment of the neuropathic bowel by electrical stimulation of the rectum. *Developmental Medicine and Child Neurology* **16**, 336.

KEMP D.R. (1966) The forgotten bladder. *British Journal of Surgery* **53**, 236.

KLAUS M.H., JERAULD R., KREGER N.C., McALPINE W., STEFFA M. & KENNELL J.H. (1972) Maternal attachment: importance of the first post-partum days. *New England Journal of Medicine* **286**, 460.

KLENERMAN L. & MERRICK M.V. (1973) Anterior sacral meningocele occurring in a family. *Journal of Bone and Joint Surgery* **55B**, 331.

KNOX E.G. (1966) Spina bifida in Birmingham. *Developmental Medicine and Child Neurology,* Supplement **13**, 14.

KNOX E.G. (1972) Anencephalus and dietary intakes. *British Journal of Preventive and Social Medicine* **26**, 219.

KOLIN I.S., SCHERZER A.L., NEW B. & GARFIELD M. (1971) Studies of the school-age child with meningomyelocele: social and emotional adaptation. *Journal of Pediatrics* **78**, 1013.

KOONTZ W.W., JR., VERNON SMITH M.J. & CURRIE R.J. (1972) External sphincterotomy in boys with meningomyelocele. *Journal of Urology* **108**, 649.

LANCET (1969) Editorial. Natural history of spina bifida. *Lancet* **ii**, 34.

LANCET (1971) Editorial. Handicapped children in normal schools. *Lancet* **ii**, 752.

LANDAUER W. (1945) Rumplessness of chicken embryos produced by the injection of insulin and other chemicals. *Journal of Experimental Zoology* **98**, 65.

LASSMAN L.P., JAMES C.C.M. & FOSTER J.B. (1968) Hydromyelia. *Journal of Neurological Sciences* **7**, 149.

LAURENCE K.M. (1964) The natural history of spina bifida cystica. *Archives of Disease in Childhood* **39**, 41.

LAURENCE K.M. (1966) The survival of untreated spina bifida cystica. *Developmental Medicine and Child Neurology,* Supplement **11**, 10.

LAURENCE K.M. (1974) Effect of early surgery for spina bifida on survival and quality of life. *Lancet* **i**, 301.

LAURENCE K.M., BLIGH A.S. & EVANS K.T. (1968) Vertebral and other abnormalities in parents and sibs of cases of spina bifida cystica and of anencephaly. *Developmental Medicine and Child Neurology,* Supplement **16**, 107.

LAURENCE K.M., CARTER C.O. & DAVID P.A. (1968) Major central nervous system malformations in South Wales. *British Journal of Preventive and Social Medicine,* **22**, 146.

LAURENCE K.M. & TEW B.J. (1971) Natural history of spina bifida cystica and cranium bifidum cysticum. *Archives of Disease in Childhood* **46**, 127.

LA VIELLE C.J. & CAMPBELL D.A. (1958) Neurofibromatosis and intrathoracic meningocele. *Radiology* **70**, 62.

LEARMONTH J.R. (1931) A contribution to the neurophysiology of the urinary bladder in man. *Brain* **54,** 147.

LEBEDEFF A. (1881) Uber die Enstehung der Anencephalie und spina bifida bei Vogeln und Menschen. *Virchows Arch. path. Anat.* **86,** 263.

LECK I. (1969) Ethnic differences in the incidence of malformations following migration. *British Journal of Preventive and Social Medicine* **23,** 166.

LECK I., RECORD R.G., MCKEOWN T. & EDWARDS J.H. (1968) The incidence of malformations in Birmingham, England 1950–1959. *Teratology* **1,** 263.

LEMIRE R.J. (1974) Embryology of the Central Nervous System. In *Scientific Foundations of Paediatrics,* ed. Davis J.A. & Dobbing J. London: Heinemann.

LESI F.E.A. (1968) A study of congenital malformations in newborn in Lagos. Ph.D. Thesis. Trinity College, Dublin.

LIGHTOWLER C.D.R. (1971) Meningomyelocele: the price of treatment. *British Medical Journal* **ii,** 385.

LINDER R. (1970) Mothers of disabled children – the value of weekly group meetings. *Developmental Medicine and Child Neurology* **12,** 202.

LISTER J. (1971) Open myelomeningocele. M.D. Thesis. University of Edinburgh.

LISTER J., COOK R.C.M. & ZACHARY R.B. (1968) Operative management of neurogenic bladder dysfunction in children: ureterostomy. *Archives of Disease in Childhood* **43,** 672.

LORBER J. (1965) The family history of spina bifida cystica. *Pediatrics* **35,** 589.

LORBER J. (1968) The results of treatment of extreme hydrocephalus. *Developmental Medicine and Child Neurology,* Supplement **16,** 21.

LORBER J. (1969a) Spina bifida. *Practitioner* **202,** 522.

LORBER J. (1969b) Ventriculo-cardiac shunts in the first week of life. *Developmental Medicine and Child Neurology,* Supplement **20,** 13.

LORBER J. (1971a) Results of treatment of myelomeningocele. An analysis of 524 unselected cases with special reference to possible selection for treatment. *Developmental Medicine and Child Neurology* **13,** 279.

LORBER J. (1971b) Medical and surgical aspects in the treatment of congenital hydrocephalus. *Neuropädiatrie* **3,** 239.

LORBER J. (1971c) What are the chances for the second generation? *Link* **1,** 10.

LORBER J. (1972) Spina bifida cystica: results of treatment of 270 consecutive cases with criteria for selection for the future. *Archives of Disease in Childhood* **47,** 854.

LORBER J. (1973a) Early results of selective treatment of spina bifida cystica. *British Medical Journal* **iv,** 201.

LORBER J. (1973b) Isosorbide in the medical treatment of infantile hydrocephalus. *Journal of Neurosurgery* **39,** 702.

LORBER J. & BRUCE A.M. (1963) Prospective controlled studies in bacterial 'meningitis' in spina bifida cystica. *Developmental Medicine and Child Neurology* **5,** 146.

LORBER J. & LYONS V.H. (1970) Arterial hypertension in children with spina bifida cystica and urinary incontinence. *Developmental Medicine and Child Neurology,* Supplement **22,** 101.

LORBER J., MENEER P.C. & ALLOTT D.C. (1967) An investigation into prophylactic treatment of urinary tract infections in infants born with spina bifida cystica. *Developmental Medicine and Child Neurology,* Supplement **15,** 30.

LORBER J. & SCHLOSS A.L. (1973) The adolescent with myelomeningocele. *Developmental Medicine and Child Neurology,* Supplement **29,** 113.

LORBER J. & SEGALL M. (1962) Bacterial meningitis in spina bifida cystica. A review of 37 cases. *Archives of Disease in Childhood* **37,** 300.

LOWE C.R., ROBERTS C.J. & LLOYD S. (1971) Malformations of the central nervous system and softness of local water supplies. *British Medical Journal* **ii,** 357.

LUTHARDT T. (1970) Bacterial infections in ventricule-atrial shunt systems. *Developmental Medicine and Child Neurology,* Supplement **22,** 105.

MCDONALD P. (1973) Malignant sacrococcygeal teratoma: report of four cases. *American Journal of Roentgenalogy Radium Therapy Nuclear Medicine* **118,** 494.

MCHAFFIE G.G. (1974) Personal communication.

MACKEITH R.C. (1973) The feelings and behaviour of parents of handicapped children. *Developmental Medicine and Child Neurology* **15,** 524.

MCKIBBIN B. (1973) The use of splintage in the management of paralytic dislocation of the hip in spina bifida cystica. *Journal of Bone and Joint Surgery* **55B,** 163.

McLAURIN R.L. & DODSON D. (1971) Infected ventriculo-atrial shunts: some principles of treatment. *Developmental Medicine and Child Neurology*, Supplement **25**, 71.

MEADOW S.R. (1973) Shunt nephritis: renal disease associated with infected ventriculo-atrial shunts. *Developmental Medicine and Child Neurology* **15**, 83.

MEDICAL RESEARCH COUNCIL (1943) Aids to the investigation of peripheral nerve injuries. *War Memorandum No. 7*. H.M.S.O., London.

MELLINS R.B., BALFOUR H.H., TURINO G.M. & WINTERS R.W. (1970) Failure of automatic control of respiration (Ondine's curse). Report of an infant born with this syndrome and a review of the literature. *Medicine* (Baltimore) **49**, 487.

MENELAUS M.B. (1971) The orthopaedic management of spina bifida cystica. Edinburgh: Livingstone.

MILHORAT T.H. (1972) Hydrocephalus and the cerebrospinal fluid. Baltimore: The Williams and Wilkins Co.

MILLER E. & SETI L. (1971) The effect of hydrocephalus on perception. *Developmental Medicine and Child Neurology*, Supplement **25**, 77.

MORGAGNI G.B. (1761) *De sedibus et causis morborum per anatomen indigatis*. Translated by B. Alexander (1769). London: Millar and Cadell.

MORLEY A.R. (1969) Laryngeal stridor. Arnold-Chiari malformation and medullary haemorrhages. *Developmental Medicine and Child Neurology* **11**, 471.

MORRICE J.J. & YOUNG D.G. (1974) Bacterial colonisation of Holter valves: a 10-year survey. *Developmental Medicine and Child Neurology*, Supplement **32**, 85.

MORTON J. (1877) Treatment of Spina Bifida. London.

MURTAGH F. & LEHMAN R. (1967) Peritoneal shunts in the management of hydrocephalus. *Journal of the American Medical Association* **202**, 1010.

MUSTARDÉ J.C. (1966) Meningomyelocele: the problems of skin cover. *British Journal of Surgery* **53**, 36.

NAGGAN L. & McMAHON B. (1967) Ethnic differences in the prevalence of anencephaly and spina bifida in Boston, Mass. *New England Journal of Medicine* **277**, 1119.

NASH D.F.E. (1956) Congenital spinal palsy. *British Medical Journal* **2**, 1333.

NASH D.F.E. (1968) Ethical and social aspects of treatment of spina bifida. *Lancet* **ii**, 827.

NASH D.F.E. (1972) Bowel management in spina bifida patients. *Proceedings of the Royal Society of Medicine* **65**, 70.

NEEL J.V. (1958) A study of major congenital defects in Japanese infants. *American Journal of Human Genetics* **10**, 398.

NELSON M.M. & FORFAR J.O. (1969) Congenital abnormalities at birth: their association in the same patient. *Developmental Medicine and Child Neurology* **11**, 3.

NERGÅRDH A., VON HEDENBERG C., HELLSTRÖM B. & ERICSSON N.O. (1974) Continence training of children with neurogenic bladder dysfunction. *Developmental Medicine and Child Neurology* **16**, 47.

NEWBIGGING P.S.K. (1834) *Spina Bifida*. Probationary Essays. Vol. VI. Royal College of Surgeons, Edinburgh.

NISHIMURA H., TAKANO K., TANIMURA T., YASUDA M. & UCHIDA T. (1966) High incidence of several malformations in the early human embryos as compared with infants. *Biologia Neonatorum* **10**, 93.

NORMAND I.C.S. & SMELLIE J.M. (1965) Prolonged maintenance chemotherapy in the management of urinary infection in childhood. *British Medical Journal* **i**, 1023.

NULSEN F.E. & BECKER D.P. (1966) Control of hydrocephalus by valve-regulated shunt. Infections and their prevention. *Clinical Neurosurgery* **14**, 256.

NULSEN F.E. & SPITZ E.B. (1951) Treatment of hydrocephalus by direct shunt from ventricle to jugular vein. *Surgical Forum* **2**, 399.

O'GRADY F. & CATTELL W.R. (1966) Kinetics of urinary tract infection. *British Journal of Urology* **38**, 149.

O'HARE J.M. (1958) Progress report in the study of congenital paraplegics. *Proceedings of Seventh Annual Clinical Paraplegia Conference*.

PARSCH K. & SCHULITZ K.P. (1972) Das spina-bifida-kind. Klinik und Rehabilitation. Stuttgart: Georg Thieme Verlag.

PARSONS J.G. (1972) Assessments of aptitudes in young people of school-leaving age handicapped by hydrocephalus or spina bifida cystica. *Developmental Medicine and Child Neurology*, Supplement **27**, 101.

PASSARGE E., TRUE C.W., SUEOKA W.T., BAUMGARTNER N.R. & KEER K.R. (1966) Malformations of the central nervous system in trisomy–18 syndrome. *Journal of Pediatrics* **69**, 771.

PATEL C.D. & MATLOUB H. (1973) Vaginal perforation as a complication of ventriculoperitoneal shunt. *Journal of Neurosurgery* **38**, 761.

PENFIELD W. & COBURN D.F. (1938) Arnold-Chiari malformation and its treatment. *Archives of Neurology and Psychiatry* **40**, 328.

PENFIELD W. & ELVIDGE A.R. (1932) Hydrocephalus and the atrophy of cerebral compression. In *Cytology and Cellular Pathology of the Nervous System*, ed. W. Penfield, vol. 3, p. 1201. New York: Hafner.

PERRIN J.C.S. & McLAURIN R.L. (1967) Infected ventriculo-atrial shunts. A method of treatment. *Journal of Neurosurgery* **27**, 21.

PILLING D. (1973) The child with spina bifida. Social, emotional and educational adjustment: an annotated bibliography. Slough: N.F.E.R. Publishing Company Ltd. for National Childrens' Bureau.

POND H.S. & TEXTER J.H. (1970) Trigonal-ileal anastomosis: experimental studies. *Journal of Urology* **103**, 746.

POTTHOFF P.C. & HEMMER R. (1969) Valve insufficiency in ventriculo-atrial shunts. *Developmental Medicine and Child Neurology*, Supplement **20**, 38.

PUDENZ R.H. (1966) The ventriculo-atrial shunt. *Journal of Neurosurgery* **5**, 601.

PUDENZ R.H., RUSSELL F.E., HURD A.M. & SHELDEN C.H. (1957) Ventriculo-auriculostomy. A technique for shunting cerebro-spinal fluid into the right auricle. *Journal of Neurosurgery* **14**, 171.

RAIMONDI A.J. & MATSUMOTO S. (1967) A simplified technique for performing the ventriculo-peritoneal shunt. Technical note. *Journal of Neurosurgery* **26**, 357.

RÁLIŠ Z.A. (1974) The role of mechanical intrauterine pressure in the pathogenesis of paralytic limb deformities. *Journal of Bone and Joint Surgery* **56B**, 383.

RÁLIŠ Z.A. (1975) Traumatising effect of breech delivery on infants with spina bifida. *Journal of Pediatrics* **87**, 613.

RECKLINGHAUSEN F.D. VON (1886) Untersuchungen über die spina bifida. *Virchow Arch. Path. Anat.* **105**, 243, 373.

RECORD R.G. & McKEOWN T. (1949) Congenital malformations of the central nervous system. *British Journal of Social Medicine* **3**, 183.

RICHARDS I.D.G., ROBERTS C.J. & LLOYD S. (1972) Area differences in prevalence of neural tube malformations in South Wales. A study of possible demographic determinants. *British Journal of Preventive and Social Medicine* **26**, 89.

RICHARDS I.D.G. & McINTOSH H.T. (1973) Spina bifida survivors and their parents: a study of problems and services. *Developmental Medicine and Child Neurology* **15**, 293.

RICHINGS J.C. & ECKSTEIN H.B. (1970) Locomotor and educational achievements of children with myelomeningocele. *Annals of Physical Medicine* **10**, 291.

RICKHAM P.P. & PENN I.A. (1965) The place of the ventriculostomy reservoir in the treatment of myelomeningocele and hydrocephalus. *Developmental Medicine and Child Neurology* **7**, 296.

RIVEILLE C. (1962) Problèmes psychologiques dans le spina-bifida paralytique. *Ann. Méd. psychiat.* **125**, 5.

ROBERTS J.B.M. (1961) Congenital anomalies of the urinary tract and their association with spina bifida. *British Journal of Urology* **33**, 309.

ROBERTS J.R. & RICKHAM P.P. (1970) Craniostenosis following Holter valve operation. *Developmental Medicine and Child Neurology*, Supplement **22**, 145.

RUBIN R.C., HOCHWALD G., LIWNICZ B., TIELL M., MIZUTANI H. & SHULMAN K. (1972) The effect of severe hydrocephalus on size and number of brain cells. *Developmental Medicine and Child Neurology*, Supplement **27**, 117.

RUSSELL D.S. (1949) Observations on the pathology of hydrocephalus. *Medical Research Council Special Report Series* **265**. London: H.M.S.O.

RUYSCH F. (1691) Observationum anatomico chirurgicarum centuria. H. & T. Boom, Amsterdam.

SANDØE E., BRYNDORF J. & GERTZ T.C. (1959) Cystometry. A new technique applying a percutaneously inserted catheter in the bladder. *Danish Medical Bulletin* **6**, 194.

SCOBIE W.G., ECKSTEIN H.B. & LONG W.J. (1970) Bowel function in myelomeningocele. *Developmental Medicine and Child Neurology*, Supplement **22**, 150.

SCOTT F.B., BRADLEY W.E. & TIMM G.W. (1974) Treatment of urinary incontinence by an implantable prosthetic urinary sphincter. *Journal of Urology* **112**, 75.

SCOTT J.E.S. (1973) Urinary diversion in children. *Archives of Disease in Childhood* **48**, 199.

SCOTT M., ROBERTS E.G.G. & TEW B. (1975) Psychosexual problems in adolescent spina bifida patients. *Developmental Medicine and Child Neurology*, Supplement **35**, 158.

SEDZIMIR C.B., ROBERTS J.R. & OCCLESHAW J.V. (1973) Massive diastematomyelia without cutaneous dysraphism. *Archives of Disease in Childhood* **48**, 400.

SEGALAS M. (1844) On the influence of traumatic lesions of the spinal cord on the genito-urinary functions. *Lancet* **2**, 99.

SELLA A., FOLTZ E.L. & SHURTLEFF D.B. (1966) A three-year developmental study of treated and untreated hydrocephalic children. *Journal of Pediatrics* **69**, 887.

SHALLAT R.F., PAWL R.P. & JERVA M.J. (1973) Significance of upward gaze palsy (Parinaud's syndrome) in hydrocephalus due to shunt malfunction. *Journal of Neurosurgery* **38**, 717.

SHARRARD W.J.W. (1962) Mechanism of paralytic deformity in spina bifida. *Developmental Medicine and Child Neurology* **4**, 310.

SHARRARD W.J.W. (1964a) The segmental innervation of the lower limb muscles in man. *Annals of the Royal College of Surgeons* **35**, 106.

SHARRARD W.J.W. (1964b) Posterior iliopsoas transplantation in the treatment of paralytic dislocation of the hip. *Journal of Bone and Joint Surgery* **46B**, 426.

SHARRARD W.J.W. (1968) Spinal osteotomy for congenital kyphosis in myelomeningocele. *Journal of Bone and Joint Surgery* **50B**, 466.

SHARRARD W.J.W. (1973) The orthopaedic surgery of spina bifida. *Clinical Orthopaedics and Related Research* **92**, 195.

SHARRARD W.J.W. & DRENNAN J.C. (1972) Osteotomy – excision of the spine for lumbar kyphosis in older children with myelomeningocele. *Journal of Bone and Joint Surgery* **54B**, 50.

SHARRARD W.J.W. & GROSFIELD L. (1968) The management of deformity and paralysis in the foot in myelomeningocele. *Journal of Bone and Joint Surgery* **50B**, 456.

SHARRARD W.J.W., ZACHARY R.B., LORBER J. & BRUCE A.M. (1963) A controlled trial of immediate and delayed closure in spina bifida cystica. *Archives of Disease in Childhood* **38**, 18.

SHURTLEFF D.B. (1973) Central nervous system infections in hydrocephalus or myelo-dysplasia. *Clinical Pediatrics* **12**, 310.

SJÖGREN I. (1968) Echoencephalographic measurement of ventricular size in children. *Developmental Medicine and Child Neurology* **10**, 145.

SMITH E.D. (1965) *Spina Bifida and Total Care of the Spinal Myelomeningocele.* Springfield, Illinois: Thomas.

SMITH E.D. (1972a) Urinary prognosis in spina bifida. *Journal of Urology* **108**, 815.

SMITH E.D. (1972b) Follow-up studies on 150 ileal conduits in children. *Journal of Pediatric Surgery* **7**, 1.

SMITH G.K. & SMITH E.D. (1973) Selection for treatment in spina bifida cystica. *British Medical Journal* **iv**, 189.

SMITH T.W.D., DUCKWORTH T. & MALTBY B. (1973) The importance of reflex function in myelomeningocele. *Developmental Medicine and Child Neurology*, Supplement **29**, 47.

SMITHELLS R.W. & CHINN E.R. (1965) Spina bifida in Liverpool. *Developmental Medicine and Child Neurology* **7**, 258.

SMYTH B.T., PIGGOT J., FORSYTHE W.I. & MERRET J.D. (1974) A controlled trial of immediate and delayed closure of myelomeningocele. *Journal of Bone and Joint Surgery* **56B**, 297.

SPERLING D.F., PATRICK J.R., ANDERSON F.M. & FYLER D.C. (1964) Cor pulmonale secondary to ventriculo-auriculostomy. *American Journal of Diseases in Childhood* **137**, 308.

STARK G.D. (1967) Treatment of ventriculitis in hydrocephalic infants: intrathecal and intraventricular use of the new penicillins. *Developmental Medicine and Child Neurology*, Supplement **15**, 36.

STARK G.D. (1968) The pathophysiology of the bladder in myelomeningocele and its correlation with the neurological picture. *Developmental Medicine and Child Neurology*, Supplement **16**, 76.

STARK G.D. (1969) Pudendal neurectomy in management of neurogenic bladder in myelomeningocele. *Archives of Disease in Childhood* **44**, 698.

STARK G.D. (1971) Neonatal assessment of the child with a myelomeningocele. *Archives of Disease in Childhood* **46**, 539.

STARK G.D. (1972a) The nature and cause of paraplegia in myelomeningocele. *Paraplegia* **9**, 219.

STARK G.D. (1972b) Cerebral oedema. *Developmental Medicine and Child Neurology* **14**, 814.

STARK G.D. (1973a) Correlative studies of bladder function in myelomeningocele. *Developmental Medicine and Child Neurology*, Supplement **29**, 55.

STARK G.D. (1973b) Spina bifida cystica. In *Textbook of Paediatrics*, Forfar and Arneil. Edinburgh: Churchill Livingstone.

STARK G.D. (1975) Myelomeningocele: the changing approach to treatment. In *Recent Advances in Paediatric Surgery*, ed. A.W. Wilkinson, 3rd Ed. London: Churchill Livingstone.

STARK G.D. & BAKER G.C.W. (1967) The neurological involvement of the lower limbs in myelomeningocele. *Developmental Medicine and Child Neurology* **9**, 732.

STARK G.D., BASSETT W.J., BAIN D.J.G. & STEWART F.I. (1975) Paediatrics in Livingston New Town. The evolution of a child health service. *British Medical Journal* **iv**, 387.

STARK G.D. & DRUMMOND M. (1970) Spina bifida as an obstetric problem. *Developmental Medicine and Child Neurology*, Supplement **22**, 157.

STARK G.D. & DRUMMOND M. (1971) The spinal cord lesion in myelomeningocele. *Developmental Medicine and Child Neurology*, Supplement **25**, 1.

STARK G.D. & DRUMMOND M. (1972) Neonatal electromyography and nerve conduction studies in myelomeningocele. *Neuropädiatrie* **3**, 409.

STARK G.D. & DRUMMOND M. (1973) Results of selective early operation in myelomeningocele. *Archives of Disease in Childhood* **48**, 676.

STARK G.D., DRUMMOND M., PONEPRASERT S. & ROBARTS F.H. (1974) Primary ventriculoperitoneal shunts in treatment of hydrocephalus associated with myelomeningocele. *Archives of Disease in Childhood* **49**, 112.

STEIN S., SCHUT L. & BORNS P. (1974) Lacunar skull deformity (Lückenschädel) and intelligence in myelomeningocele. *Journal of Neurosurgery* **41**, 10.

STRACH E.H. (1972) The spring implant operation: a preliminary report. *Developmental Medicine and Child Neurology*, Supplement **27**, 121.

STEVENSON A.C., JOHNSTON H.A., STEWART M.I.P. & GOLDING A.R. (1966) Congenital malformations. A report of a study of a series of consecutive births in 24 centres. *Bulletin of the World Health Organisation* Supplement **34**.

SUSSET J.G., TAGUSHI Y., DE DOMINICO I. & MACKINNON K.J. (1966) Hydronephrosis and hydroureter in ileal conduit urinary diversion. *Canadian Journal of Surgery* **9**, 141.

SUTOW W.W. & PRYDE A.W. (1956) Incidence of spina bifida occulta in relationship to age. *American Journal of Diseases of Children* **91**, 211.

SWISHER L.P. & PINSKER E.J. (1971) The language characteristics of hyperverbal, hydrocephalic children. *Developmental Medicine and Child Neurology* **13**, 746.

TAVERNER D. & SMIDDY F.G. (1959) An electromyographic study of the normal function of the external anal sphincter and pelvic diaphragm. *Diseases of Colon and Rectum* **2**, 153.

TEW B.J. & LAURENCE K.M. (1972) The ability and attainments of spina bifida patients born in South Wales between 1956–1962. *Developmental Medicine and Child Neurology*, Supplement **27**, 124.

TEW B.J. & LAURENCE K.M. (1973) Mothers, brothers and sisters of patients with spina bifida. *Developmental Medicine and Child Neurology*, Supplement **29**, 69.

TEW B.J. & LAURENCE K.M. (1975) The effects of hydrocephalus on intelligence, visual perception and school attainment. *Developmental Medicine and Child Neurology*, Supplement **35**, 129.

TEW B.J., PAYNE H. & LAURENCE K.M. (1974) Must a family with a handicapped child be a handicapped family? *Developmental Medicine and Child Neurology*, Supplement **32**, 95.

THOMAS G.G., SHAPIRO S.R. & JOHNSTON J.H. (1975) Ureteral re-implantation in children with neurogenic vesical dysfunction. *Developmental Medicine and Child Neurology*, Supplement **35**, 159.

THOMAS M. & HOPKINS J.M. (1971) A study of the renal tract from birth in children with myelomeningocele. *Developmental Medicine and Child Neurology*, Supplement **25**, 96.

THIERRY A., ARGHIMBAUD J-P., FISCHER G., FRE'DEL M. & MANSUY L. (1969) La méningocèle sacrée antérieure. *Neurochirurgie* **15**, 389.

THIERSH J.B. (1952) Therapeutic abortions with a folic acid antagonist, 4-amino-pteroyl-glutamic acid administered by the oral route. *American Journal of Obstetrics and Gynaecology* **63**, 1298.

TILL K. (1969) Spinal Dysraphism: a study of congenital malformations of the lower back. *Journal of Bone and Joint Surgery* **51B**, 415.

TRYFONAS G. (1973) Three spina bifida defects in one child. *Journal of Pediatric Surgery* **8**, 75–6.

TSHIRGI R.D., FROST R.W. & TAYLOR J.L. (1954) Inhibition of cerebrospinal fluid formation by a carbonic anhydrase inhibitor (Diamox). *Proceedings of the Society for Experimental Biological Medicine* **87**, 373.

TSINGOGLOU S. & ECKSTEIN H.B. (1970) Cardiac perforation by Holter shunts. *Developmental Medicine and Child Neurology*, Supplement **22**, 170.

TSUCHIDA Y., SATO T. & ISHIDA M. (1972) Radiographic anorectal function study in myelomeningocele. *Journal of Paediatric Surgery* **7**, 50.

TUCKEY L., PARFIT J. & TUCKEY B. (1973) Handicapped school leavers. Slough: N.F.E.R. Publishing Company Ltd.

TULPIUS N. (1652) Observationes medicae. Amsterdam.

TÜNTE W. (1971) Fortpflanzungs fähigkeit, Heiratshäofigkeit und Zahl und Beschaffenheit der Nachkommen bei Patienten mit Spina bifida aperta. *Humangenetik*, **13**, 43.

UEMATSU S. & WALKER A.E. (1967) Ultrasonic determination of the size of the cerebral ventricular system. *Neurology* (Mineap.) **17**, 81.

VARIEND S. & EMERY J.L. (1973) The weight of the cerebellum in children with myelomeningocele. *Developmental Medicine and Child Neurology*, Supplement **29**, 77.

VARIEND S. & EMERY J.L. (1974) The pathology of the central lobes of the cerebellum in children with myelomeningocele. *Developmental Medicine and Child Neurology*, Supplement **32**, 99.

VILLOT, CARDINAL JEAN (1970) L'Osservatore Romano, Oct. 12–13.

WALD N.J., BROCK D.J.H. & BONNAR J. (1974) Prenatal diagnosis of spina bifida and anencephaly by maternal serum alpha-fetoprotein measurement. A controlled study. *Lancet* **i**, 765.

WALKER G.F. (1968) The orthopaedics of myelomeningocele in infancy. *Hospital Medicine* **2**, 900.

WALKER J.H., THOMAS M. & RUSSELL I.T. (1971) Spina bifida – and the parents. *Developmental Medicine and Child Neurology* **13**, 462.

WALLACE S.J. (1973) The effect of upper limb function on mobility of children with myelomeningocele. *Developmental Medicine and Child Neurology*, Supplement **29**, 84.

WEALTHALL S.R. (1973) An investigation of the factors involved in regulating ventricular size and the production of hydrocephalus. *Developmental Medicine and Child Neurology*, Supplement **29**, 1.

WEALTHALL S.R., TODD J.H. & BALL C. (1973) The role of A-scope encephalography in childhood hydrocephalus. *Developmental Medicine and Child Neurology*, Supplement **29**, 92.

WEALTHALL S.R., WHITTAKER G.E. & GREENWOOD N. (1974) The relationship of apnoea and stridor in spina bifida to other unexplained infant deaths. *Developmental Medicine and Child Neurology*, Supplement **32**, 107.

WELBOURN H. (1975) Spina bifida children attending ordinary schools. *British Medical Journal* **i**, 142.

WELLER R.O., WISNIEWSKI H., ISHI N., SHULMAN K. & TERRY R.D. (1969) Brain tissue damage in hydrocephalus. *Developmental Medicine and Child Neurology*, Supplement **20**, 1.

WEST K.A. (1967) Correlations between ultrasonic and roentgenologic findings in infantile hydrocephalus. *Acta Paediatrica Scandinavica* **56**, 27.

WHITE J.J., SUZUKI H., EL SHAFIE M., KUMAR A.P.M., HELLER J.A. & SCHNAUFER L.

(1972) A physiologic rationale for the management of neurologic rectal incontinence in children. *Pediatrics* **49**, 888.

WILCOCK A.R. & EMERY J.L. (1970) Deformities of the renal tract in children with myelomeningocele and hydrocephalus, compared with those of children showing no such central nervous system deformities. *British Journal of Urology* **42**, 152.

. WILLIAMS B. (1971) Further thoughts on the valvular action of the Arnold-Chiari malformation. *Developmental Medicine and Child Neurology,* Supplement **25**, 105.

WILLIS T.A. (1931) The separate neural arch. *Journal of Bone and Joint Surgery* **13**, 709.

WILSON C.B. & BERTAN V. (1966) Perforation of the bowel complicating peritoneal shunt for hydrocephalus: review of two cases. *American Surgery* **32**, 601.

· WINBERG J. (1973) Urinary tract infections in infants and children. In *Textbook of Paediatrics,* Forfar and Arneil Eds. Edinburgh: Churchill Livingstone.

WINTER R.B., MOE J.W. & EILERS V.E. (1968) Congenital scoliosis: a study of 234 patients treated and untreated. *Journal of Bone and Joint Surgery* **50A,** 1.

WOODBURN M.F. (1974) Social implications of spina bifida – a study in South-East Scotland. Scottish Spina Bifida Association, Edinburgh.

YAKOVLEV P.I. (1947) Paraplegias of hydrocephalics (a clinical note and interpretation). *American Journal of Mental Deficiency* **51**, 561.

ZACHARY R.B. (1968) Ethical and social aspects of treatment of spina bifida. *Lancet* **ii,** 274.

ZACHARY R.B. & LISTER J. (1972) Conservative management of the neurogenic bladder. Chapter 5 in *Problems in Paediatric Urology,* Johnston, J.H. and Scholtmeijer, R.J. Eds. Amsterdam: Excerpta Medica, 1972.

ZACHARY R.B. & SHARRARD W.J.W. (1967) Spinal dysraphism. *Postgraduate Medical Journal* **43**, Supplement **1**, 731.

Index